facials and skincare

in essence

facials and skincare

in essence

Helen McGuinness

Series Editor: Nicola Jenkins

Hodder Arnold

A MEMBER OF THE HODDER HEADLINE GROUP

The author and publishers would like to thank the following for the use of photographs in this volume:

p.2 (left) akg-images/Erich Lessing, (right) Peter Stuart/Rex Features; p.4 Matt Baron/BEI/Rex Features; p.32 (left) Lauren Shear/Science Photo Library; p.32 (right), p.33 (left) © Mediscan; p.33 (right), p.37 (left) Dr. H.C. Robinson/Science Photo Library; p.34 (left), p.40 Wellcome Photo Library; p.34 (right), p.35 (bottom left and right), p.36, p.38 (top left), p.39, p.42 (top and bottom) Dr. P. Marazzi/Science Photo Library; p.35 (top left) CNRI/Science Photo Library, p.37; (top right) Dr. Chris Hale/Science Photo Library; p.38 (bottom left) CNRI/Science Photo Library, (bottom right) BSIP/Science Photo Library; p.48 PurestockX; p.54 Mauro Fermariello/Science Photo Library; p.70 © Paul Vozdic/The Image Bank/Getty Images; p.71 © Matthias Clamer/Stone+/Getty Images; p.86 Collin UK, Pevonia UK Ltd, Dermatologica and Decléor; p.115 Sorisa; p.120, 123 Xavier G. Cosmetic Skin Clinic.

Commissioned photographs © by Carl Drury.
With thanks to our model Minna, and to Images Model Agency.

Orders: please contact Bookpoint Ltd, 130 Milton Park, Abingdon, Oxon OX14 4SB. Telephone: (44) 01235 827720. Fax: (44) 01235 400454. Lines are open from 9.00 – 5.00, Monday to Saturday, with a 24 hour message answering service. You can also order through our website www.hoddereducation.co.uk

British Library Cataloguing in Publication Data
A catalogue record for this title is available from the British Library

ISBN 978 0 340 92693 2

First Published 2007
Impression number   10 9 8 7 6 5 4 3 2
Year   2012 2011 2010 2009 2008 2007

Copyright © 2007 Helen McGuinness

Cover photo © Image Shop/Corbis
Typeset by Servis Filmsetting Ltd, Manchester
Printed in Malaysia for Hodder Arnold, an imprint of Hodder Education and a member of the Hodder Headline Group, an Hachette Livre UK Company, 338 Euston Road, London NW1 3BH

contents

foreword

Since I carried out my original beauty therapy training over 20 years ago, the skincare industry has developed significantly, which has meant that beauty therapists need to be very knowledgeable about the skin, and all matters relating to the skin, including innovations and new developments.

In this book I therefore wanted to create a wealth of knowledge that took the reader beyond the basics of skincare to help them to broaden their continuing professional development.

I hope that this book will bring inspiration to students, professionals and teachers of facial massage and skincare.

As an additional study resource, free Multiple Choice Questions and answers are available for downloading at www.hoddereducation.co.uk → Search → Facials.

Helen J. McGuinness

acknowledgements

I am deeply grateful to the following people who have helped me realise one of my ambitions in writing this book, which is uniquely written to address the needs of the facial/skincare specialist.

Firstly to Mark, my husband, who has, as always, provided tremendous love and much-needed encouragement, as well as support in helping me to organise and format the book. He should also be acknowledged for his tireless efforts to help me source research information for the history of skincare in Chapter 1.

To our beautiful daughter Grace (who also happens to have beautiful skin!), who has provided me with lots of inspiration, love and laughter in the writing of this book.

To my parents Roy and Val, who have always provided love, along with the support and encouragement of my writing.

To my dearest friend Dee Chase for her constant love, support and positive encouragement, and especially for always having faith and belief in my abilities.

To another dear friend, and seasoned skincare professional, Sue Muir, who kindly read the whole manuscript (even when feeling unwell!), suggested some very valuable additions to the text, and whose opinion I have always valued.

To Heather Mole, Regional Verifier for VTCT, for kindly providing excellent resource information to assist me with the writing of Chapter 1.

To Dr Xavier Goodarzian MD (Hons) MRCGP Dip Clin Derm (London), and Martin McKenzie MA (Hons) MICB for kindly assisting me with information for Chapter 8.

Finally to all the staff and students at the Holistic Training Centre who have, sometimes unknowingly, provided me with valuable knowledge and experience to assist me in the writing of this book.

introduction

A facial is one of the most popular treatments because it is beneficial in improving skin condition and is extremely relaxing to receive. Once considered a luxury, regular facials and skincare maintenance treatments are now regarded as more of a necessity. Having good skin can make clients look healthy, and improving the appearance, texture and look of the skin is an important factor for most clients, regardless of age.

During the last decade the skincare market has developed into a multi-million pound business as awareness of skincare and well-being has become more prevalent. The emphasis in the 21st century has been on promoting health of the skin from the inside out and on combating the effects of age, stress and the environment. There has been a great interest in the development of medical aesthetics, involving the integration of cosmetic and surgical procedures with aesthetic treatments in the pursuit of skin rejuvenation.

With the emergence of skincare products containing more potent and scientific ingredients, there are more efficient methods of treating a wide range of skin problems. Clients in a salon today will present a range of challenges to the therapist, including acne, rosacea, ageing skin, sun-damaged skin and sensitivity, to name but a few. In order to meet the needs of the client, facial skincare specialists need to be knowledgeable about the skin, products and a range of applications.

Due to the ever-evolving nature of skin therapy, there are always development opportunities for therapists to extend their skills 'beyond the basics'. The importance of continuing one's education cannot be over-emphasised, as clients demand more and more from their skincare programmes. Depending on your client market this may mean learning advanced manual techniques to increase the effectiveness of your facials, or may mean training in the techniques of more advanced skincare products or equipment.

The history of skincare

Modern skincare is rooted in ancient civilisation; our ancestors as far back as biblical times used skin preparations as a means of maintaining health and beauty.

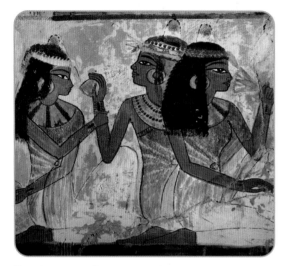

Egyptian image of beauty

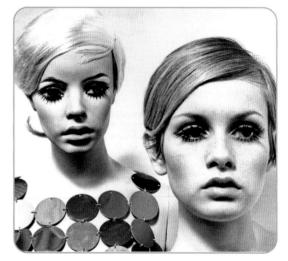

Image of beauty in the 1960s

Mesolithic Period

- Skin softened with castor oil and grease.
- Plant dye tattoos.

Biblical Times

- Skin softening lotions made from olive oil and spices.

Egyptians

- Cleopatra writes a beauty book and bathes in milk (alphahydroxy acids; AHAs) to soften skin.
- Exfoliants, depilatories, anti-wrinkle creams created.
- Egyptian anti-wrinkle cream recipe: one teaspoon of sweet almond oil to two drops of essential oil of frankincense.
- Cosmetics for both sexes.
- Moisturisers and oils used to protect skin.
- Face packs made from barley and crushed sesame seeds.
- Soap made from soapwort, animal fats and fragrant oils.

Greeks

- Recipe for cold cream using beeswax, olive oil and rose water.
- Recommended finely ground garden snails as a moisturiser.

Romans

- Steam therapy, body scrubs and massage therapies on offer at Roman baths (built over hot sulphur springs).
- Rich oils used on skin.
- Hair dyes: mineral quicklime, walnut oil.
- Milk, bread and wine used for facials.
- Other facials used cornflour and milk.

Middle Ages

- Eyebrows plucked.
- Face masks using ground asparagus roots and goat's milk.
- Perfumes and antiseptics from essential oils.
- Hair gel from swallow's droppings and lizard tallow.

Renaissance

- Lead used to whiten faces.
- Beauty spots to cover blemishes.
- Hair dye from saffron or sulphur.
- Toothpowders from sage, nettles and powdered clay.
- Perfume used to cover body odour.

Elizabethan

- White lead face paint (mixed with vinegar).
- Hair tonic and lightener from oil of vitrol (sulphuric acid) and rhubarb juice.
- Whisked egg whites used to tighten and glaze the skin.
- A popular base for rouge and skin creams was bear's grease.
- Iridescent eye shadow made of ground mother of pearl.
- Red wine, ass's milk, rainwater and urine used as facial cleaners.

Nicholas Culpeper: Culpeper's Complete Herbal 1600s

- Broom stalks to cleanse the skin.
- Oatmeal boiled with vinegar to treat spots and pimples.
- Wheat bread soaked in rose water to soothe tired eyes.
- Woodbine ointment for sunburn.

Victorian

- 1825 *The Art of Beauty*: advice included erasing wrinkles by becoming overweight and using belladonna juice to enlarge the pupils.
- Beauty masks and face packs made from many ingredients that are still used such as honey, eggs, oatmeal, milk, fruit, and vegetables.
- No skin creams or cosmetics were used in polite society. Only a dot of eau de cologne was respectable.
- Baths were a mixture of hot water and milk with herbs such as flax seeds to soften the skin.

continued

20th and 21st Centuries

- 1908 Elizabeth Arden originated concept of a 'beauty cream'; developed natural-based skin-care products.
- 1946 Estee Lauder launched her own company with a jar of skin cream developed by an uncle who was a chemist.
- 1955 Lancôme launched *Oceane* product line containing pure seaweed enriched with algae and trace elements.
- 1960s Women began to use facial moisturisers; cold creams, such as Ponds, Nivea or Astral, for cleansing.
- 1962 Society of Beauticians founded.
- 1970s – Examining body took the name International Health and Beauty Council (IHBC).
- 1970s and 1980s Manufacturers introduced a wider range of products for the skin.
- 1980s First NVQs (National Vocational Qualifications) introduced by The Health and Beauty Therapy Industry Training Board.
- 1990s Skincare linked to well-being: products based on botanicals, essential oils, aromatic extracts, antioxidants and vitamins.
- 2000s Wide choice of professional skincare products available in salons and spas around the world.
- Medical aesthetics developing.
- Men's skincare becomes popular.

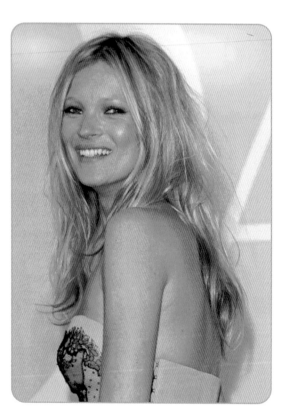

Modern day image of beauty

anatomy and physiology

A comprehensive knowledge of the structure and functions of the skin will help facial therapists treat clients more effectively and carry out facial treatments to a safe and competent level. Linking skin structure and function to the client's skin condition will facilitate an accurate skin analysis and ultimately offer the correct choice of products and treatment.

In order to understand the skin's structure and functions, it is important to examine the structure and activities of cells, which are the building blocks of the layers of the skin (the epidermis and dermis).

Cells

The principal job of cells is to manufacture protein which then becomes the building material for making tissues. Cells are fundamental to the life of skin and all other body organs in that they process food, oxygen, water and waste for the body. Each cell is a microscopically small unit, surrounded by a delicate membrane.

Cell membrane

Cell membrane is a fine membrane that encloses the cell and protects its contents. It is made up of lipids (fats) and protein, which allow selective permeability: it has the capacity to selectively control the inward and outward movement of molecules into and out of the cell. Oxygen, nutrients, hormones and proteins are taken into the cell as needed and cellular waste such as carbon dioxide passes out through the membrane.

Protruding from the cell membrane are the receptor sites, whose function is to receive messages from hormones and other chemical messengers made by other cells. When a chemical comes into contact with a specific receptor site, a message is sent to the cell to carry out its specific function. A good example of this is the sebaceous glands: sebum production is stimulated by male hormones that are received by the receptor sites in the sebaceous gland cells.

As well as governing the exchange of nutrients and waste materials, the membrane also maintains the shape of the cell.

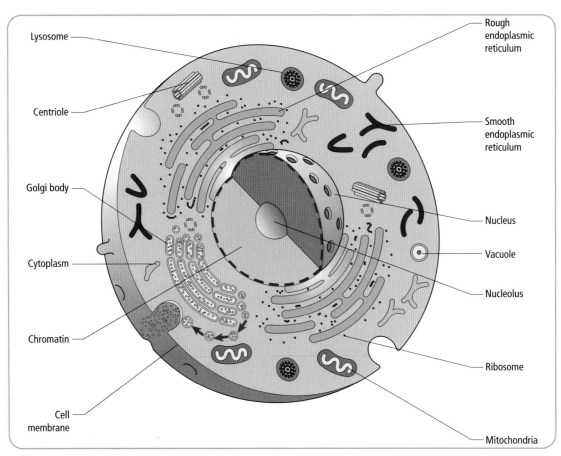

Structure of a cell

Cytoplasm

Cytoplasm is the gel-like substance that is enclosed by the cell membrane. It is made up of water and other substances, and contains the nucleus and the small cellular structures called organelles. The cytoplasm allows the organelles to move around in the cell and therefore most cellular metabolism occurs within the cytoplasm of the cell.

Mitochondria

Mitochondria are oval shaped organelles that lie within the cytoplasm. The mitochondria provide most of a cell's ATP (adenosine triphosphate), which is a compound that stores the energy needed by the cell.

The work of the mitochondria is assisted by enzymes, which are proteins that speed up chemical changes. By means of cellular respiration, the mitochondria provide the energy which powers the cell's activities.

Endoplasmic reticulum

This is a series of membranes continuous with the cell membrane. It can be thought of as an intracellular transport system, allowing movement of materials from one part of the cell to another. It links the cell membrane with the nuclear membrane and therefore assists movement of materials within and out of the cell.

The endoplasmic reticulum contains enzymes and participates in the synthesis of proteins, carbohydrates and lipids. It stores material, transports substances inside the cell and detoxifies harmful agents. Some endoplasmic reticulum appears smooth, while some appears rough due to the presence of ribosomes.

Ribosomes

Ribosomes are tiny organelles made up of ribonucleic acid (RNA) and protein. They may be fixed to the walls of the endoplasmic reticulum (known as rough ER), or may float freely in the cytoplasm.

Their function is to manufacture proteins for use within the cell, and also to produce other proteins that are exported outside the cell.

Lysosome

These are round sacs present in the cytoplasm. They contain powerful enzymes, which are capable of digesting proteins. Their function is to destroy any part of the cell that is worn out so that it can be eliminated – this is known as lysis.

Vacuole

These are empty spaces within the cytoplasm. They contain waste materials or secretions formed by the cytoplasm and are used for temporary storage, transportation or digestive purposes in different kinds of cells.

Golgi body/apparatus

This is a collection of flattened sacs within the cytoplasm. The golgi apparatus is typically located near the nucleus and attached to the endoplasmic reticulum. It stores the protein manufactured in the endoplasmic reticulum and later transports it out of the cell.

Nucleus

The nucleus is the largest organelle in the cytoplasm and is the control centre of the cell, regulating the cell's functions and directing nearly all metabolic activities. The nucleus governs the specialised work performed by the cell and the cell's own growth, repair and reproduction.

The chromatin is the substance inside the nucleus that contains the genetic material. The information on the cell's characteristics is stored in DNA (deoxyribonucleic acid). The DNA strands are found in threadlike structures known as chromosomes which carry the genetic information in the form of genes. The nucleus of a human cell contains 46 chromosomes, 23 of which are of maternal and 23 of which are of paternal origin. Each chromosome can create an exact copy of itself through cell division and each new cell formed contains a full set of chromosomes.

Inside the nucleus is a dense spherical structure called a nucleolus, which contains ribonucleic acid (RNA) structures that form ribosomes.

The nucleus is surrounded by a perforated outer membrane called the nuclear membrane; materials move across it to and from the cytoplasm.

Note DNA determines many characteristics of the skin such as colouring, oiliness, dryness, sensitivity, acne and also the ageing process.

Cell growth and reproduction

Cells have the ability to create new cells to replace those which have worn out or become damaged. Skin cells reproduce by dividing into two identical daughter cells, in a process known as mitosis. Cell growth and reproduction rely on favourable conditions such as an adequate supply of food, oxygen, water, suitable temperatures and the ability to eliminate waste.

If conditions become unfavourable for the skin, such as smoking, sun damage and air pollution, cell function will become impaired and skin cells may subsequently be destroyed.

Structure of the skin

Having knowledge of the function of the skin cell layers is fundamental to understanding the process of cell renewal in the skin, and to understanding the process of product penetration.

There are two main layers of the skin:

- The epidermis, which is the outer thinner layer.
- The dermis, which is the inner thicker layer.

Below the dermis is the subcutaneous layer which attaches to organs and tissues.

Although the skin is technically a single organ, the two main layers do have different structures and functions.

The epidermis

The epidermis is the most superficial layer of the skin and consists of five layers of cells:

- The basal cell layer (stratum germinativum) – innermost layer.
- The prickle cell layer (stratum spinosum).
- The granular layer (stratum granulosum).
- The clear layer (stratum lucidum).
- The horny layer (stratum corneum) – outermost layer.

In most areas of the body the epidermis is approximately 35–50 micrometres thick. It is thicker on the palms and soles of the feet (up to several millimetres), and thinner around the eye (approximately 20 micrometres).

Note The basal cell layer holds approximately 80 per cent water and each subsequent layer holds less so that the horny layer holds about 15 per cent. The skin's capacity to retain water decreases with age, making the ageing skin more vulnerable to dehydration and wrinkles.

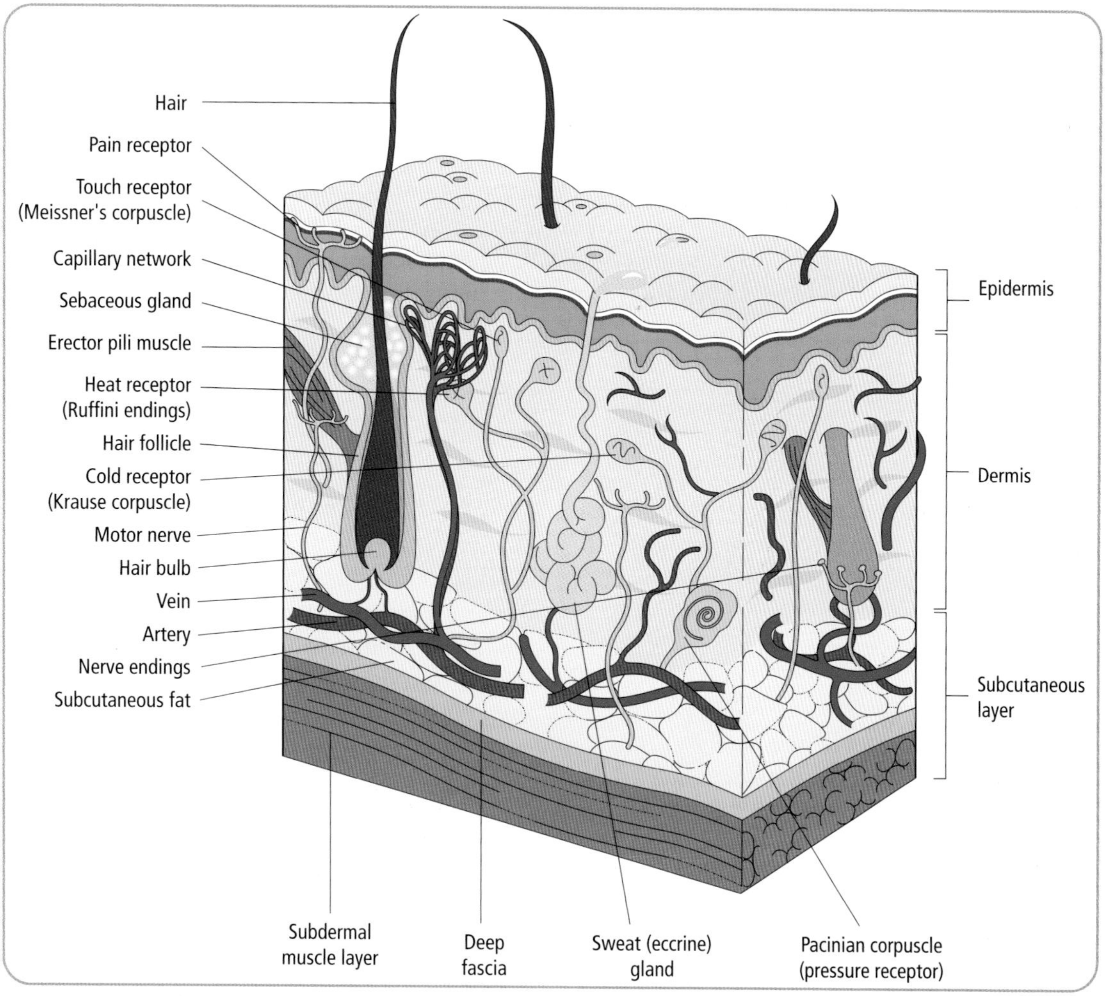
Hair
Pain receptor
Touch receptor
(Meissner's corpuscle)
Capillary network
Sebaceous gland
Erector pili muscle
Heat receptor
(Ruffini endings)
Hair follicle
Cold receptor
(Krause corpuscle)
Motor nerve
Hair bulb
Vein
Artery
Nerve endings
Subcutaneous fat
Epidermis
Dermis
Subcutaneous
layer
Subdermal
muscle layer
Deep
fascia
Sweat (eccrine)
gland
Pacinian corpuscle
(pressure receptor)

Structure of the skin

Functions of the epidermis

The epidermis has three primary functions:

- Protecting the body from the external environment, particularly the sun.
- Preventing excessive water loss from the body.
- Protecting the body from infection.

The basal cell layer (stratum germinativum)

This consists of a single layer of column cells on a basement membrane and is where cell regeneration takes place. The basal cells within this layer are continuously producing new cells that constantly divide. As new cells are formed, they push adjacent cells towards the skin's surface.

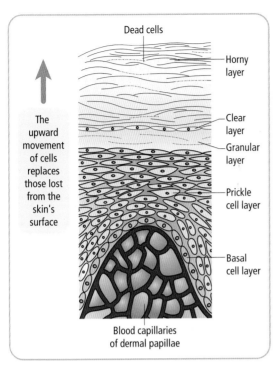

Layers of the epidermis

Approximately 95 per cent of the cells within the epidermis are keratinocytes, which produce a protein substance called keratin. Keratin is what makes the epidermal cells more resilient and protective as they are pushed towards the skin's surface.

At intervals between the column cells, which divide to reproduce, are the large star-shaped cells called melanocytes, which form the pigment melanin, the skin's main colouring agent. This layer also contains tactile (Merkel) discs that are sensitive to touch.

Prickle cell layer (stratum spinosum)

This is the thickest layer of the epidermis. It is known as the prickle cell layer because each of the rounded cells contained within it has short

projections which make contact with the neighbouring cells and give it a prickly appearance. The tiny hairlike structures on the prickle cells will eventually become desmosomes, which are small disc shaped attachments that provide strength and integrity by holding the upper level of epidermal cells together. The cells of this layer are living and are therefore capable of dividing by the process mitosis.

This layer also includes Langerhans cells which set up an immune response to foreign bodies.

Granular layer (stratum granulosum)

This layer consists of distinctly shaped cells that resemble granules, which are filled with keratin and produce intercellular lipids (the substances that fill the spaces between the upper epidermal cells) from structures called lamellar bodies.

These lipids help form a strong cement-like structure to prevent the absorption of harmful substances by the skin and help maintain hydration of the lower layers. These cells create an appearance of a wall of bricks (cells) and mortar (lipids).

Note The cells in the prickle cell layer make special fats called sphingolipids. When these cells reach the horny layer these lipids play an important role in the retention of moisture in the skin.

Clear layer (stratum lucidum)

This layer consists of transparent cells which permit light to pass through. The cells in the clear layer are filled with a substance called eleidin, which is produced from keratohyalin and is involved in the keratinisation process.

Note The clear layer is considered to be an important transitional stage in the development of the horny layer of the epidermis.

The clear layer is very thin in facial skin, but thick on the soles of the feet and the palms of the hands, and is generally absent in hairy skin.

Horny layer (stratum corneum)

This is the most superficial outer layer, consisting of dead, flattened keratinocytes, now known as corneocytes. The horny layer is the end result of the change that occurs when new live cells produced in the basal layer are pushed upwards by newer cells until they reach the surface where they dry out and are continually shed; this process is known as desquamation.

The horny layer forms a waterproof covering for the skin and helps to prevent the penetration of bacteria. It is this layer that is directly affected by the external environment.

Note The horny layer plays a key role in helping to contain moisture in the rest of the skin and in regulating the natural moisture flow from the deeper layers to be lost in evaporation from the skin surface. This natural moisture flow is known as transepidermal water loss (TEWL).

Without adequate retained moisture skin can become dry and unhealthy. Under normal conditions, up to 15 per cent of the horny layer consists of water, which is vital to enable the stratum corneum to work. The natural functions of the skin do not work as efficiently when the horny layer contains less than 10 per cent of water, and it becomes dry.

Life span of the epidermal cells

In normal skin, it takes approximately 28–30 days for a cell produced by the basal layer to move through the epidermis to the surface. The rate of regeneration is partly determined by the rate at which the outer layer is being desquamated. With age this process is greatly reduced and by the age of 50 it is said to take about 37 days to complete the same process.

When the cells of the horny layer are lost quickly (for instance due to skin injury or sunburn) the process speeds up as the cells are replaced more quickly from below. Removing the outer layers of the skin with a chemical peel will also speed up replacement.

Note An essential factor in beautiful skin is the healthy metabolism of keratinocytes. If the keratinocyte formation is not functioning properly it cannot generate an aesthetically pleasing horny layer. A healthy balance of all the essential elements (water, lipids, etc.) is needed to ensure that the health of the keratinocytes is not impaired.

Keratinisation

Keratinisation refers to the process that skin cells undergo when they change from living cells with a nucleus to dead cells without a nucleus.

The dermis

The dermis lies below the epidermis and can be as much as 3000 micrometres thick. It contains several types of tissue that provide a supporting framework to the skin, as well as blood vessels, nerves, hair roots, sweat and sebaceous glands.

11

Skin layer	Keratinisation process
Basal cell	New living cells begin migrating upwards towards the horny layer. They are held together and to the dermis by desmosomes.
Prickle cell	Chemical changes takes place in the upper cells of this layer and keratinisation begins. It is here the keratinocyte has a major role to play in skin barrier defence.
Granular	As the cells move up this layer, further changes to the keratinocyte occur. They become less flexible and more granular in appearance and the keratin within the cell hardens, thereby completing the keratinisation process.
Clear	The keratinocyte has almost reached its final destination by the time it reaches the clear layer.
Horny	The keratinocytes become corneocytes (dead skin cells) and the desmosomes begin to dissolve in preparation for desquamation.

The functions of the dermis include:

- Providing nourishment to the epidermis.
- Removing waste products from the epidermis.
- Giving a supporting framework to the tissues by providing shape and holding all its structures together.
- Contributing to skin colour.

The dermis has two layers: a superficial papillary layer and a deeper reticular layer.

The papillary layer

The superficial papillary layer is made up of fatty connective tissue and is connected to the underside of the epidermis by cone-shaped projections called dermal papillae which contain nerve endings and a network of blood and lymphatic capillaries. The fine network of capillaries brings oxygen and nutrients to the skin and carries the waste away.

Note The key function of the papillary layer of the dermis is to provide vital nourishment to the living layers of the epidermis above.

The reticular layer

The deeper reticular layer is formed of tough fibrous connective tissue which helps to give the skin strength and elasticity, and helps to support and hold all structures in place.

The protein collagen, which accounts for about 75 per cent of the weight of the dermis and is organised in bundles running horizontally throughout the dermis, is buried in a jelly-like material called the ground substance. Collagen gives the skin its resilience and elasticity.

The collagen bundles are held together by elastic fibres running through the dermis made from a protein called elastin, which makes up less than 5 per cent of the skin's weight. Both collagen and elastin fibres are made by cells called fibroblasts which are found throughout the dermis.

An important substance that forms part of the tissue surrounding the collagen and elastin fibres is hyaluronic acid. This has the ability to attract and bind hundreds of times its weight in water and in this way maintains the moisture content and plumps the skin's tissues.

The glycoproteins found in the ground substance of the dermis are capable of holding large amounts of water and maintaining its accumulation.

Note Damage to collagen and elastin fibres as they break down is the primary cause of ageing and wrinkles. Similarly, when the amount of hyaluronic acid and glycoproteins produced in the skin decreases, the skin becomes less resilient and loses elasticity.

In addition to fibroblasts, other cells present in the dermis include:

- Mast cells which secrete histamine causing dilation of blood vessels, bringing blood to the area.
- Phagocytic cells (macrophages), which are white blood cells able to travel around the dermis destroying foreign matter and bacteria.

Blood supply

The dermis is well supplied with capillary blood vessels bringing nutrients and oxygen to the germinating cells in the basal cell layer of the epidermis and removing waste products from them.

Arteries carry oxygenated blood to the skin via arterioles and these enter the dermis from below and branch into a network of capillaries around active or growing structures. These capillary networks form in the dermal papillae to provide the basal cell layer of the epidermis with food and oxygen. They also surround the sweat glands and erector pili muscles.

The capillary networks drain into venules (small veins) which carry the deoxygenated blood away from the skin and remove waste products.

Lymphatic vessels

There are numerous lymphatic vessels in the dermis forming a network facilitating the removal of waste from the skin's tissue. The lymphatic vessels in the skin generally follow the course of veins and are found around the dermal papillae, glands and hair follicles.

Nerves
Sensory nerves

There are several different types of sensory nerve endings in the skin.

- Touch.
- Pressure.
- Pain.
- Temperature.

The sensory nerve endings are also called receptors because they are receiving information.

Touch receptors

These receptors are located immediately below the epidermis. They are stimulated by light pressure on the skin which enables a person to distinguish between different textures such as rough, smooth, hard and soft.

Pressure receptors

These receptors are situated beneath the dermis and are stimulated by heavy pressure.

Pain receptors

These receptors consist of branched nerve endings in the epidermis and dermis. They are quite evenly distributed throughout the skin and are important in that they provide a warning signal of damage or injury in the body.

Temperature receptors

There are separate hot and cold receptors in the skin that are stimulated by sudden changes in temperature.

The dermis also has motor nerve endings, which relay impulses from the brain and are responsible for the dilation and constriction of blood vessels, the secretion of perspiration from the sweat glands and the contraction of the erector pili muscles attached to hair follicles.

The subcutaneous layer

This is a thick layer of connective tissue found below the dermis. The adipose tissue, which contains fat cells, helps support delicate structures such as blood vessels and nerve endings. It also cushions the dermis from underlying tissues such as muscles and bones.

The areolar tissue in this layer contains collagen, elastin and reticular fibres, which make it elastic and flexible and bind the skin to the muscles. It contains the major arteries and veins which supply the skin and form a network throughout the dermis. The fat cells contained within this layer help to insulate the body by reducing heat loss. Below the subcutaneous layer lies the subdermal muscle layer.

> Note As we grow older, the amount of fat starts to decrease in the subcutaneous layer and eventually results in a bonier look to the facial contours.

Appendages of the skin
Hair

Hair is an appendage of the skin which grows from a sac-like depression in the epidermis called a hair follicle. Hair grows all over the body, with the exception of the palms of the hands and the soles of the feet. The primary function of hair is in physical protection, for example, the hair on the scalp provides partial shading from the sun's rays, and the hairs in the nostrils, eyelashes and eyebrows provide protection from foreign particles.

The structure of a hair
The hair is composed mainly of the protein keratin and is therefore a dead structure.

The hair is divided into three parts:

- Hair shaft – the part of the hair that lies above the surface of the skin.
- Hair root – the part of the hair found below the skin.
- Hair bulb – the enlarged part at the base of the hair root.

Internally the hair has three layers which all develop from the matrix, the active growing part of the hair.

The erector pili muscle is a small smooth muscle attached at an angle to the base of a hair follicle and makes the hair stand erect in response to cold.

Sweat glands

There are two types of sweat glands. The majority are eccrine glands, which are simple coiled tubular glands that open directly on to the surface of the skin. There are several million of them distributed over the surface of the skin although they are most numerous in the palms of the hands and the soles of the feet. Their function is to regulate body temperature and help eliminate waste products. The sweat they secrete is controlled by the sympathetic nervous system.

The other type of sweat glands are apocrine glands; these are connected with hair follicles and are found in the genital and underarm regions. They produce a fatty secretion; breakdown of the secretion by bacteria leads to body odour.

Sebaceous glands

These glands are found all over the body, except for the soles of the feet and the palms of the hands. They are more numerous on the scalp, face, chest and back.

Sebaceous glands commonly open into a hair follicle but some open on to the skin surface. They produce an oily substance called sebum which contains fats, cholesterol and cellular debris.

Sebum coats the surface of the skin and the hair shafts, preventing excess water loss and lubricating and softening the horny layer of the epidermis and the hair.

> Note A facial stimulates the circulation and so facilitates cell nutrition and regeneration and increases elimination of waste from the skin's tissues. Massage can loosen dead keratinised cells blocking the pores so the blood flows more freely to feed the skin.

The functions of the skin

The skin has several important functions, in that it offers protection, temperature regulation and waste removal, as well as providing us with a sense of touch.

Protection

- The skin acts like a physical barrier protecting the underlying tissues from abrasion. Keratin provides protection by waterproofing the skin's surface, helping to keep water in and out.
- The skin also provides limited protection from ultraviolet radiation through specialised cells called melanocytes found in the basal cell layer of the epidermis.
- The skin's acidic secretions (sweat and sebum), known as the *acid mantle*, act as a barrier against foreign agents such as bacteria and viruses.
- Fat cells in the subcutaneous layer of the skin help protect bones and major organs from injury.

> Note The mantle of the skin is acidic and varies in pH between 4.5 and 6.2 on the pH scale. The pH scale measures the concentration of hydrogen ions in a substance and determines whether a product is acid or alkaline. It is important for therapists to consider variations in pH levels of substances, as products with either a high or low pH value may be harmful to the skin and may cause damage to the barrier function, resulting in irritation.

Temperature regulation

The skin helps to regulate body temperature in the following ways:

- In cool environments, the blood capillaries near the skin surface contract, to keep warm blood away from the surface of the skin and closer to major organs.
- The erector pili muscles raise the hairs and trap air next to the skin.

15

- The adipose tissue in the dermis and the subcutaneous layer helps to insulate the body against heat loss.
- When the body is too warm, the blood capillaries dilate to allow warm blood to flow near to the surface of the skin, in order to cool the body.
- The evaporation of sweat from the surface of the skin also cools the body.

Sensitivity

The skin is considered as an extension of the nervous system. It is very sensitive to various stimuli due to its many sensory nerve endings which can detect changes in temperature and pressure, and register pain.

Excretion

The skin functions as a mini-excretory system, eliminating waste through perspiration. The eccrine glands of the skin produce sweat, which helps to remove some waste materials such as urea, uric acid, ammonia and lactic acid.

Storage

The skin also acts as a storage depot for fat and water. About 15 per cent of the body's fluids are stored in the subcutaneous layer.

Absorption

The skin has limited absorption properties. The epidermis can absorb fat soluble substances such as oxygen, carbon dioxide, fat soluble vitamins, steroids and small amounts of water.

> Note The skin is capable of absorbing small particles of substances such as essential oils due to the fact that they contain fat and water soluble particles.

Vitamin D production

Modified cholesterol molecules in the skin are converted by the ultraviolet rays in sunlight to vitamin D. This is then absorbed by the body for the maintenance of bones and to aid the absorption of calcium and phosphorus in the diet.

Bones related to facial structure

It is important for facial therapists to study the bones of the head, neck and shoulders in order to understand how, along with the muscles and fatty tissue, they provide shape and contour to the facial skin.

The skull

The skull consists of 22 bones:

- 8 bones that make up the skull or cranium
- 14 forming the facial skeleton.

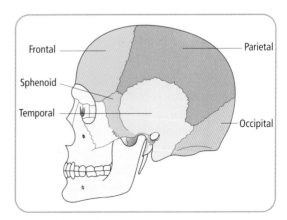

Bones of the skull

The bones of the skull

Frontal	Forms the anterior part of the roof of the skull.
Parietal (x2)	Form the upper sides of the skull and the back of the roof of the skull.
Temporal (x2)	Form the sides of the skull below the parietal bones and above and around the ears. The temporal bone contributes to part of the cheekbone via the zygomatic arch.
Sphenoid	Located in front of the temporal bone and serves as a bridge between the cranium and the facial bones.
Occipital	Forms the back of the skull.
Ethmoid	Forms part of the wall of the orbit, the roof of the nasal cavity and part of the nasal septum.

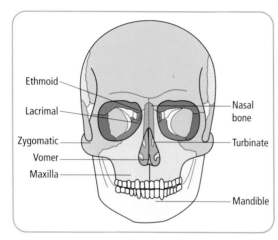

Bones of the face

Bones of the face

Maxillae (x2)	Largest bones of the face; they form the upper jaw and support the upper teeth.
Mandible	The only moveable bone of the skull; forms the lower jaw and supports the lower teeth.
Zygomatic (x2)	These are the most prominent of the facial bones; they form the cheekbones.
Nasal (x2)	These small bones form the bridge of the nose.
Lacrimal (x2)	The smallest of the facial bones, located close to the medial part of the orbital cavity.
Turbinate (x2)	Layers of bone located either side of the outer walls of the nasal cavities.
Vomer	Single bone at the back of the nasal septum.
Palatine (x2)	L-shaped bones which form the anterior part of the roof of the mouth.

Bones of the neck, chest and shoulder girdle

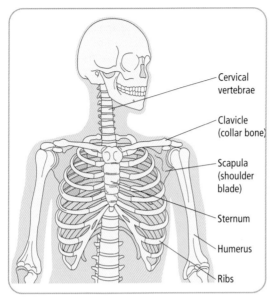

Bones of the neck, chest and shoulder girdle

Labels on figure:
- Cervical vertebrae
- Clavicle (collar bone)
- Scapula (shoulder blade)
- Sternum
- Humerus
- Ribs

The shoulder girdle

The shoulder girdle connects the upper limbs with the thorax and consists of four bones:

- Two clavicles.
- Two scapulae.

The humerus

The humerus is the long bone of the upper arm. The head of the humerus articulates with the scapula, forming the shoulder joint.

The sternum

The sternum is commonly referred to as the breast bone and is a flat bone lying just beneath the skin in the centre of the chest.

The neck

The neck comprises of seven bones known as the cervical vertebrae.

Muscles of the head, neck and shoulders

The muscles of the head, neck and shoulders are made up of voluntary muscle tissue, which is under conscious control.

As our muscles are in constant use throughout life, over a period of years sagging, lines, wrinkles and dropped contours appear in the skin. These conditions are generally caused by one or more of the following factors:

- Repetitive facial movement, as a result of constant facial expression (for example, frowning).
- Deterioration in collagen and elastin.
- Depletion of the skin's fatty layer, due to ageing and gravity.

- Muscle sagging due to the loosening of facial ligaments that hold the muscle in place.

Muscles that affect the facial contours include:

- The frontalis muscle, which causes forehead frown lines on the forehead.
- The orbicularis oculi muscle, which causes overhanging lids and bags under the eyes.
- The orbicularis oris muscle, which causes vertical lines around the mouth.
- The platysma muscle, which causes a crepy neck and dropped facial contours.

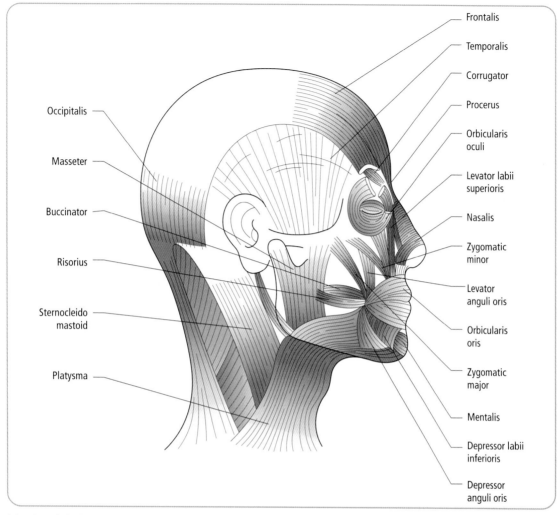

Muscles of the head and neck

Muscles of the head and neck

Muscle	Position	Action
Frontalis	Extends over front of skull and width of forehead.	Wrinkles forehead and raises eyebrows.
Occipitalis	At back of head; attaches to occipital bone and skin of scalp.	Moves scalp backwards.
Temporalis	Fan-shaped muscle situated on side of skull above and in front of ear.	Raises lower jaw when chewing.
Orbicularis oculi	Surrounds eye.	Closes eye; compresses lacrimal gland, aiding flow of tears.
Orbicularis oris	Surrounds mouth.	Closes mouth.

19

Muscles of the head and neck *continued*

Muscle	Position	Action
Corrugator	Located between eyebrows; attached to frontalis muscle and inner edge of eyebrow.	Brings eyebrows together.
Procerus	Located between eyebrows; attached to nasal bones and frontalis muscle.	Draws eyebrows inwards.
Nasalis	Located at the sides of the nose.	Dilates and compresses the nostrils.
Zygomatic major and minor (zygomaticus)	Lies in cheek area, extending from zygomatic bone to angle of mouth.	Draws angle of mouth upward and laterally.
Levator labii superioris	Located towards inner cheek beside the nose.	Raises upper lip and corner of mouth.
Levator anguli oris	From maxilla (upper jaw) to angle of mouth.	Elevation of angle of mouth.
Depressor anguli oris	From mandible (lower jaw) to angle of mouth.	Depression of angle of mouth.
Depressor labii inferioris	From mandible to midline of lower lip.	Depression of lower lip.
Risorius	Triangular-shaped muscle lying horizontally on cheek, joining at corners of mouth.	Pulls corner of mouth sideways and upwards.
Buccinator	Main muscle of cheek, attached to both upper and lower jaw.	Helps hold food in contact with teeth when chewing and compresses cheek.
Mentalis	Radiates from lower lip over centre of chin.	Elevates lower lip and wrinkles skin of chin.
Masseter	Thick, flattened, superficial muscle extending downwards from zygomatic arch to mandible.	Raises jaw and exerts pressure on teeth when chewing.
Sternocleidomastoid	Long muscle that lies obliquely across each side of neck.	When working together they flex the neck (pull chin down towards chest) and when working individually, they rotate head to opposite side.
Platysma	Superficial neck muscle that extends from chest up either side of neck to chin.	Depresses lower jaw and lower lip.

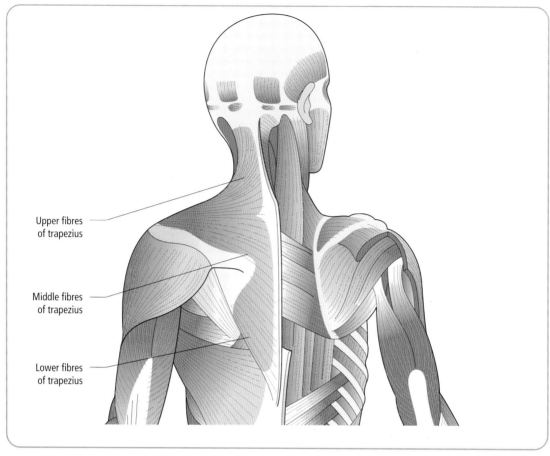

Upper fibres
of trapezius

Middle fibres
of trapezius

Lower fibres
of trapezius

Muscles of the shoulder (posterior)

Muscles of the shoulder (posterior and anterior)

Muscle	Position	Action
Trapezius (posterior)	Large triangular shaped muscle in upper back that extends horizontally from base of skull (occipital bone) and cervical and thoracic vertebrae to scapula.	Upper fibres raise shoulder girdle; middle fibres pull scapula towards vertebral column; lower fibres draw scapula and shoulder. When trapezius position fixed by other muscles, it can pull head backwards or to one side.
Deltoid (posterior)	Thick triangular muscle capping top of humerus and shoulder.	Abducts arm, draws arm backwards and forwards.
Pectoralis major (anterior)	Thick fan-shaped muscle covering anterior surface of upper chest.	Adducts arm, medially (inwardly) rotates arm.
Pectoralis minor (anterior)	Thin muscle that lies beneath pectoralis major.	Draws the shoulder downwards and forwards.

facials and skincare in essence

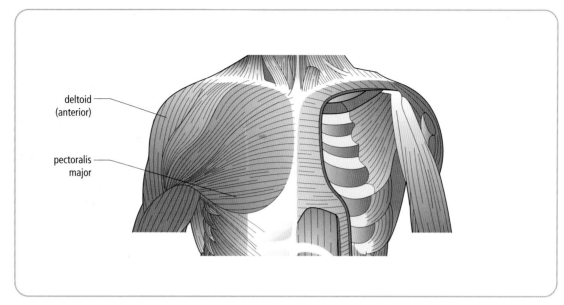

deltoid
(anterior)

pectoralis
major

Muscles of the shoulder (anterior)

Blood

Blood, pumped around the body by the heart, is the transport system which delivers and removes vital ingredients needed by the cells.

Arteries, veins and capillaries are the vessels that carry the blood to its destination. Oxygenated blood flows from the heart through the arteries and deoxygenated blood flows back to the heart through the veins. Capillaries are tiny vessels which form a network entering cell spaces to allow delivery of oxygenated blood (rich in nutrients) and removal of deoxygenated blood (full of waste products).

Blood flow to the face and head

Arteries of the head

Blood is pumped to the head via the common carotid artery, which has two branches.

- The internal carotid artery passes through the temporal bone of the skull behind the ear and takes blood to the brain.

- The external carotid artery divides into facial, temporal and occipital arteries which supply blood to the skin and muscles of the face, side and back of the head.

Veins of the head

Blood is collected from the scalp by the facial, occipital and posterior veins, which run alongside similarly named arteries. These join to form an external jugular vein behind and below the ear on both sides.

- The external jugular veins go down the neck and enter the subclavian veins.

- The internal jugular veins, which bring blood from the brain, go down on either side of the neck and enter the subclavian veins.

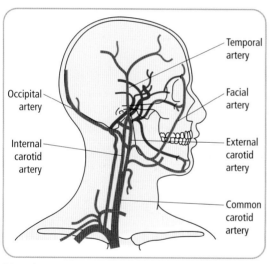

Blood flow to the head and neck

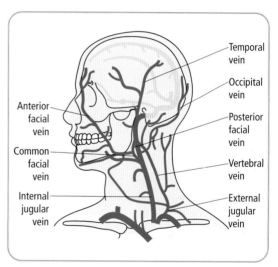

Venous drainage from the head and neck

Blood circulation and skin and muscle condition

Massage increases the blood flow to the area, which is seen as an erythema or reddening of the skin.

Facial massage has the effect of:

- Speeding up the flow of blood through the veins and helping carry away metabolic waste.
- Increasing the delivery of fresh blood to the area, bringing oxygen and nutrients to the cells, so helping cell repair and growth.
- Creating warmth by the increase in blood flow (relaxing the client).
- Improving muscle efficiency and response due to the increased oxygen and nutrients delivered to the muscle tissue.
- Improving the skin's appearance (will look softer and brighter) due to increase of nutrients to the cells.
- Removing waste products to give a toned and more relaxed appearance to the muscles.

Lymph

Lymph is the body's secondary circulatory system for collecting waste products. It carries the waste from the tissues that the blood is unable to take. The fluid that is left behind in the tissues in known as lymph and once it is collected by the lymphatic system it is emptied back into the blood system via the subclavian veins in the upper chest. The removal of lymph from the tissue spaces prevents the tissues from becoming clogged and swollen.

Lymphatic drainage of the head and neck

The main groups of lymphatic nodes relating to the head and neck

Lymphatic nodes	Position	Areas lymph drained from
Cervical (deep)	Deep within the neck, located along path of the larger blood vessels (carotid artery and internal jugular vein).	Larynx, oesophagus, posterior of scalp and neck, superficial part of chest and arm.
Cervical (superficial)	Located at side of neck, over sternomastoid muscle.	Lower part of ear and the cheek region.
Submandibular	Beneath mandible.	Chin, lips, nose, cheeks and tongue.
Occipital	At base of skull.	Back of scalp and upper part of neck.
Mastoid	Behind ear in region of mastoid process.	Skin of ear and temporal region of scalp.
Parotid	At angle of the jaw.	Drains nose, eyelids and ear.

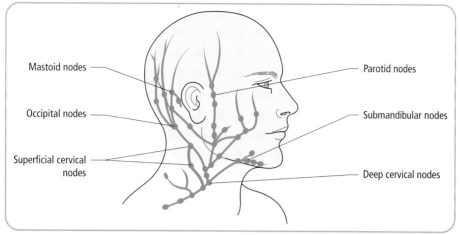

Mastoid nodes

Occipital nodes

Superficial cervical nodes

Parotid nodes

Submandibular nodes

Deep cervical nodes

Lymphatic nodes of the head and neck

The benefits of massage and the lymphatic system

Facial massage can have a very positive effect on assisting lymphatic flow, as well as skin and muscle function. The effects are as follows:

- Massage stimulates the flow of lymph, so accelerating the removal of toxins and fluid from the area.

- General swelling and puffiness can be reduced due to increased drainage of fluids from the tissues.

- Increased absorption of waste matter aids cell renewal (skin will appear softer and smoother).

- Relaxation of muscles will allow lymphatic drainage to work more efficiently (as lymphatic system does not have a pump, it relies on muscles for efficient flow and drainage).

Nerve supply to the head and neck

The nervous system transmits messages from one part of the body to the other, and consists of the network of nerve cells, or neurones.

Motor nerves carry impulses from the brain to a muscle or gland, in order to create an action or movement. For instance, when a muscle receives impulses from a motor nerve, a movement is produced. Motor nerve endings supply the muscles that produce facial expressions and move the eyes, neck and lower jaw.

Sensory nerves are widely distributed in the skin and give us sensations of touch, enabling us to distinguish between sensations of heat, cold and pain, as well as differences between light and deep pressure.

Cranial nerves

The cranial nerves connect directly to the brain. Between them, they provide a nerve supply to sensory organs, muscles and skin of the head and neck. Some of the nerves are mixed, containing both motor and sensory nerves, while others are either sensory or motor. The nerves significant to facial

25

treatments include the 5th, 7th and 11th cranial nerves.

5th cranial nerve: trigeminal

A mixed nerve that conducts impulses to and from several areas in the face and neck. It also controls the muscles of mastication (the masseter, the temporalis and the pterygoids). It has three main branches:

- The ophthalmic branch carries sensations from the eye, nasal cavity, and skin of forehead, upper eyelid, eyebrow and part of the nose.
- The maxillary branch carries sensations from the lower eyelid, upper lip, gums, teeth, cheek, nose, palate and part of the pharynx.
- The mandibular branch carries sensations from the lower gums, teeth, lips, palate and part of the tongue.

7th cranial nerve: facial

A mixed nerve that conducts impulses to and from several areas in the face and neck. It is responsible for facial expressions and branches to various muscles:

- The temporal branch supplies the muscles of the forehead and eyebrows.
- The zygomatic branch supplies the muscles of the eyes and nose.
- The buccal branch supplies the muscles of the cheek, upper lip and sides of the face.
- The mandibular branch supplies the muscles of the lower lip and chin.
- The cervical branch supplies the platysma muscle of the neck.

11th cranial nerve: accessory

Functions primarily as a motor nerve, innervating muscles in the neck and upper back (such as the trapezius and the sternomastoid), as well as muscles of the palate, pharynx and larynx.

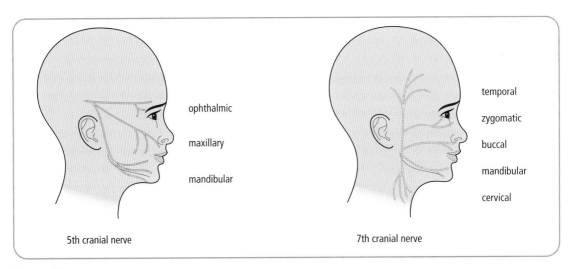

ophthalmic

maxillary

mandibular

5th cranial nerve

temporal

zygomatic

buccal

mandibular

cervical

7th cranial nerve

The cranial nerves

FAQs: Anatomy and physiology

I have read that the skin is the largest organ in the body. Exactly how large is it?

In the average adult, the skin measures approximately 2 square metres. It weighs around 9 pounds and makes up about 7 per cent of total body weight!

What keeps the skin firm and smooth?

The intercellular lipids between the epidermal cells are responsible for hydration, epidermal firmness and smoothness. They protect against transepidermal water loss, which can result in dehydration.

What is meant by the 'barrier function' of the skin?

It refers to the protective barrier supplied by the horny layer (stratum corneum) of the epidermis and the intercellular cement. This helps to protect against dehydration of the epidermis and exposure to irritating substances.

Is it true that facial muscles should be toned and exercised in order to delay ageing?

It may be possible to help a sagging neck and jaw line with appropriate exercises, however exercising muscles of the upper face will in fact increase the muscle action in that area and lead to a significant increase in the number of lines around the eyes, forehead and mouth. Botox works so effectively because it paralyses the muscles that increase lines and wrinkles.

skin diseases and disorders

Many common minor skin disorders such as comedones and mild acne are within the scope of the therapist and can benefit from regular facial treatment but some skin conditions require medical treatment. Facial therapists need to be knowledgeable about skin diseases and disorders in order to be able to recognise which require precautions, which are contraindicated in a facial treatment, and which need to be referred to another practitioner such as a GP, dermatologist, or cosmetic surgeon.

Dermatology is the branch of science that deals with the skin and its disorders. Some conditions benefit from both aesthetic and medical treatment; it is therefore not surprising that aestheticians and dermatologists are now working in close liaison with one another.

Dermatological terms

Cyst	Abnormal sac containing liquid or a semi-solid substance.
Erythema	Reddening of skin due to the dilation of blood capillaries just below the epidermis.
Fissure	Crack in the epidermis exposing the dermis.
Keloid	Overgrowth of an existing scar. The surface may be smooth, shiny or ridged. The onset is gradual, due to an accumulation of or increase in collagen in the immediate area. Colour varies from red, fading to pink and white.
Lesion	Structural change in the tissues caused by damage or injury.
Macule	Small flat patch of increased pigmentation or discoloration, e.g., a freckle.
Nodule	Solid bump that may be felt under the skin. Usually larger than 1 cm in size; may or may not be visible.
Papule	Small raised elevation on the skin, less than 1 cm in diameter, which may be red in colour.
Pustule	Infected papule which has a head with a pus-filled centre.

Dermatological terms *continued*

Scar	Mark formed from replacement tissue during wound healing. Scars may be raised (hypertrophic), rough and pitted (ice pick) or fibrous and lumpy (keloid). Scar tissue may appear smooth and shiny or form a depression in the surface.
Sebaceous cyst	Round, nodular lesion with smooth shiny surface which develops from a sebaceous gland. Usually found on face, neck, scalp and back. Situated in the dermis. Vary in size from 5–50 mm. Cause unknown. Client should be referred to GP, who may recommend surgical removal.
Telangiecstasis	Term for dilated capillaries, where there is persistent vasodilation. Usually caused by extremes of temperature and overstimulation of the tissues, although sensitive and fair skins are more susceptible.
Tumour	Formed by an overgrowth of cells. Can be benign or malignant. Tumours are lumpy and, even when they cannot be seen, they can be felt beneath the surface of the skin.
Ulcer	Break or open sore in the skin extending to all its layers.
Vesicles	Small sac-like blisters. A bulla is a vesicle larger than 0.5 cm, commonly called a blister.
Weal	Raised area of skin containing fluid, white in the centre with red edge. Seen in the condition urticaria.
Xanthoma	Buff-coloured/yellowish growth, slightly raised from the skin's surface; appears at the inner corner of the eye; texture similar to chamois leather. May be removed surgically.

Skin diseases and disorders

Although facial therapists are not qualified to diagnose a skin disorder or signs of disease in the skin, it is vital that they are able to recognise whether a client may be safely and effectively offered a facial treatment with no ill effects, such as the condition worsening or cross-infection. If the client presents with a condition that is beyond the scope of a facial treatment, it is both ethical and professional for a facial therapist to advise the client to visit a GP or a dermatologist.

Allergic reaction

An allergic reaction occurs when the body is hypersensitive to a particular allergen. When irritated by an allergen, the body produces histamine in the skin, as part of the body's defence or immune system.

The effects of different allergens are diverse. For instance, certain cosmetics and chemicals can cause rashes and irritation in the skin,

> Note In the case of a client with a nut allergy, care needs to be taken to ensure nut-based ingredients (which are common in lots of skincare products) are avoided.

allergens such as pollen, fur, feathers, mould and dust can cause asthma and hay fever.

If severe, allergies may result in anaphylactic shock, which can include rashes, swelling of the lips and throat, difficulty breathing and a rapid fall in blood pressure and loss of consciousness.

Note Although immediate reactions are more likely with skincare products, constant exposure to a particular ingredient or product can also cause the body to develop an allergy. This can be confusing to a client who may not understand that the product they have been using for years is suddenly responsible for a reaction.

In the case of a client experiencing a rash or severe redness or burning through the use of a product, the appropriate action is to remove all traces of the product immediately from the skin and apply cool, wet compresses to soothe the skin.

It is advisable for the client to discontinue all use of cosmetic products (preferably including make-up) until the reaction has stopped and all symptoms of the allergy have gone. Then clients should use products one by one on the skin, each day adding another product to see if the offending product or ingredient may be identified. In the event of a severe allergic reaction, advise the client to seek medical advice.

Acne vulgaris

A chronic inflammatory disorder of the sebaceous glands which leads to the overproduction of sebum. It involves the face, back and chest and is characterised by the presence of greasy, oily skin with enlarged pores, inflammation in and around the sebaceous glands, papules, pustules and in more severe cases cysts and scars.

Acne vulgaris is primarily androgen-induced and appears most frequently at puberty. Although commonly associated with teenage and adolescent skin, it can affect a person at different stages of life.

Typical stages of acne development

Acne starts to develop when an increase in hormone production (commonly at puberty) stimulates the sebaceous glands.

Excess sebum production causes additional cell build up in the follicles, which become comedones (plugs of sebum and dead cells).

The blocked follicle opening results in inflammation, irritation and formation of papules.

The blockage of sebum and dead skin cells prevents oxygen reaching the bottom of the follicle and hence bacteria forms. The infected papules become pustules.

The bacteria excrete an inflammatory fatty acid by-product which eventually blocks the follicle completely.

The skin forms hardened tissue to prevent the spread of bacteria, creating cysts.

The damage to the collagen and elastin in the dermis can lead to depressed and raised scars. The scars resulting from cysts are called ice-pick scars.

Note The scientific name of the bacteria that cause acne vulgaris is *proprionibacterium acnes*. These bacteria are anaerobic: they do not need oxygen to survive and grow. Although these bacteria are present in all follicles in small numbers, the oxygen provided in an open follicle prevents them from reproducing in large numbers. However, once the follicle is blocked, the oxygen cannot reach them and they multiply rapidly, feeding on the sebum produced by the overactive sebaceous glands.

There are four different grades of acne vulgaris, the grade being dependent on the severity of the disorder.

Grade I Acne	Presence of a few papules and pustules, minor breakout. Mainly open comedones present, with some closed comedones. Grade 1 acne is typical in a teenager just beginning puberty.
Grade II Acne	Greater incidence of papules and pustules, presence of many closed comedones and more open comedones.
Grade III Acne	Skin appears very red and inflamed, with many papules and pustules present.
Grade IV Acne	Cysts present with comedones, papules, pustules. Skin appears inflamed.

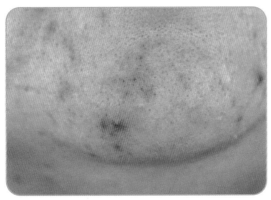

Light acne vulgaris
Presence of a few papules and pustules, minor breakout; mainly open comedones present, with some closed comedones.

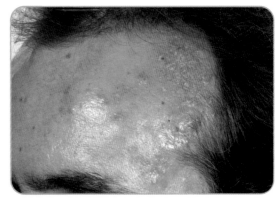

Severe acne vulgaris
Skin appears very red and inflamed, with many papules and pustules present.

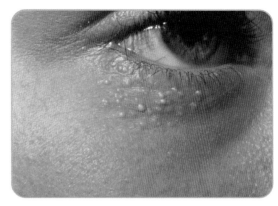

Milia

Comedones

A collection of sebum, keratinised cells and wastes which accumulate at the entrance of a hair follicle. An open comedone is a 'blackhead' contained within the follicle, whereas a closed comedone is a small bump just beneath the skin's surface.

Note Comedones are a form of skin blockage and may be released manually or with the use of a comedone extractor (see Chapter 7, page 103).

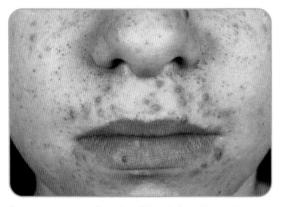

Open comedones (blackheads) and closed comedones (red raised areas)

Milia

Milia are tiny epidermal cysts found just under the surface of the skin, usually on the cheeks and around the eye area. Often called whiteheads, they appear as pearly, white, hard nodules under the skin. They contain sebaceous secretions and a build up of dead cells trapped in a blind duct with no surface opening.

More common in dry skins, milia are often formed after a skin trauma (such as sunburn) or surgical procedure (dermabrasion, chemical peels or laser resurfacing).

Note Milia may be removed with a sterile microlance. (See Chapter, 7 page 103.)

Seborrhoea

Seborrhoea is defined as an excessive secretion of sebum by the sebaceous glands. The glands appear enlarged and the skin appears greasy, especially on the nose and the centre zone of the face. Seborrhoea can resemble acne in that there may be swellings and breakout.

One of the main differences between acne and seborrhoea is that in seborrhoea the increased oil production is often accompanied by scaly, greasy-looking thickened skin, especially on the scalp.

Seborrhoea is common where there is a high incidence of sebaceous glands (for instance the scalp and the sides of the nose). It can occur at any age, but is common in infancy (when it is called 'cradle cap') and at puberty.

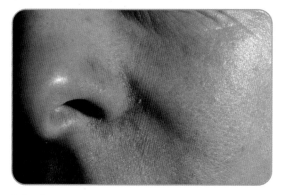

Seborrhoea

Note Depending on the severity, clients with seborrhoea may need to be referred to their medical practitioner for topical medication to help clear the condition.

Inflammatory skin disorders

Note In the case of an inflammatory skin condition care should be taken to avoid any form of stimulation (through product or treatment method) that may increase or worsen inflammation. If there is severe inflammation and the skin is broken, or there are any signs of infection, then treatment would be avoided and the client referred to their GP.

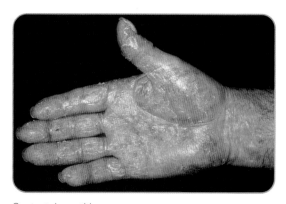

Contact dermatitis

Blepharitis

An inflammation of the eyelid, which appears red and sore. It can be caused by bacterial infection, seborrhoeic dermatitis or meibomian gland dysfunction.

Contact dermatitis

Dermatitis literally means inflammation of the skin. Contact dermatitis is caused by a primary irritant which causes the skin to become red, dry and inflamed. Substances which are likely to cause this reaction include acids, alkalis, solvent, perfumes, lanolin, detergent and nickel. There may be skin infection as well.

Eczema

A mild to chronic inflammatory skin condition characterised by itchiness, redness and the presence of small blisters that may be dry or weep if the surface is scratched. Eczema

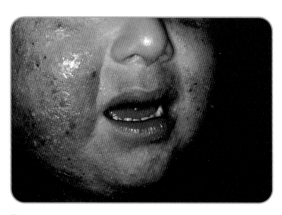

Eczema

is non-contagious: the cause may be genetic or due to internal and external influences. It can cause scaly and thickened skin, mainly at flexures, e.g. cubital area of the elbows and the back of the knees.

Systemic lupus erythematosus (SLE)

This is a chronic inflammatory disease of connective tissue affecting the skin and various internal organs. It is an autoimmune disease. It is typically characterised by a red scaly rash affecting the nose and cheeks. Other symptoms include joint pain, hair loss, and swelling of the feet and fingers.

A form of lupus which primarily affects the skin is discoid lupus erythematosus (DLE), where the skin forms round, firm lesions with red raised bumps around the hair follicles. All forms of lupus are aggravated by sun exposure.

> Note A client with lupus should be referred to their GP. Lupus is not contagious, and with the appropriate medical advice, skincare treatments may be offered. Care to avoid stimulating products and/or treatments and any of the more aggressive forms of treatment should be taken. This condition has similar needs to a sensitive skin type.

Psoriasis

A chronic inflammatory skin condition. Psoriasis may be recognised as the development of well-defined red plaques, varying in size and shape, covered by white or silvery scales. The most commonly affected sites are the face, elbows, knees, nails, chest and abdomen. Psoriasis can also affect the scalp, joints and nails. Psoriasis is aggravated by stress and trauma but is improved by exposure to sunlight.

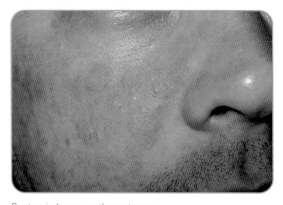

Systemic lupus erythematosus

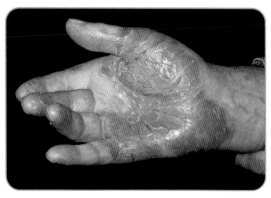

Psoriasis

Rosacea

A chronic inflammatory disease of the face in which the skin appears abnormally red, usually occurring in adults after the age of 40, but can begin as early as age 20.

The onset is gradual and begins with what first seems like a tendency to blush easily, a red complexion or an extreme sensitivity to cosmetic products. The redness appears in a characteristic butterfly pattern across the nose and cheeks and may be accompanied by dry, flaky patches. As the condition progresses there may be papules and pustules present yet rosacea is rarely accompanied by comedones. As many of the symptoms of rosacea can look like those of acne, it is a condition that is often misdiagnosed.

Many clients will develop stinging or burning sensations and the skin will often feel tight. Sometimes this progresses to the point that everything the client uses on their face stings, burns, and irritates.

Aggravating factors of rosacea include hot, spicy foods, hot drinks, alcohol, menopause, the elements and stress. It is important to avoid

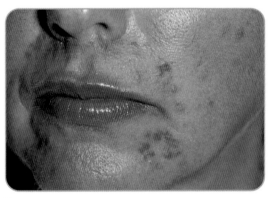

Rosacea

products that are harsh, abrasive, fragranced and heavy, and to avoid excessive extraction, steam or a very stimulating massage.

> Note Clients with rosacea should be referred to a dermatologist for diagnosis and management. If the right medication is given, along with the correct skincare treatment, it can help avoid a flaring up and worsening of the condition.

Seborrhoeic dermatitis

This is a mild to chronic inflammatory disease of those hairy areas well supplied with sebaceous glands. Common sites are the scalp, face, axilla and groin. The skin may appear to have a grey tinge or may be dirty yellow in colour. Clinical signs include slight redness, scaling and dandruff in the eyebrows.

Urticaria

Also known as 'hives'. In this condition lesions appear rapidly and disappear within minutes or gradually over a number of hours. The clinical signs are the development of red weals which may later become white. The area becomes itchy or may sting.

There are a number of causes of urticaria, some of which are an allergic reaction, e.g. to strawberries, shellfish, penicillin, house dust and pet fur. Other causes include stress and sensitivity to light, heat or cold.

Infectious skin conditions

> Note In the case of an infectious skin condition, no facial treatment can be carried out until all signs of infection have ceased; this is to prevent cross-infection and to avoid the condition spreading and/or worsening.

Bacterial infections of the skin

Boil

A boil begins as a small inflamed nodule which forms a pocket of bacteria around the base of a hair follicle, or a break in the skin.

Conjunctivitis

This is a bacterial infection following irritation of the conjunctiva of the eye. In this condition the inner eyelid and eyeball appear red and sore and there may be pus-like discharge from the eye. The infection spreads by contact with the secretions from the eye of the infected person.

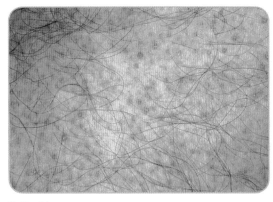

Folliculitis

Folliculitis (ingrowing hairs)

This is common amongst men and usually occurs when the mouth of a hair follicle becomes blocked and the trapped hair grows back on itself, causing a bacterial infection.

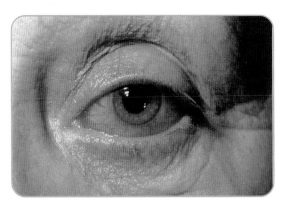

Conjunctivitis

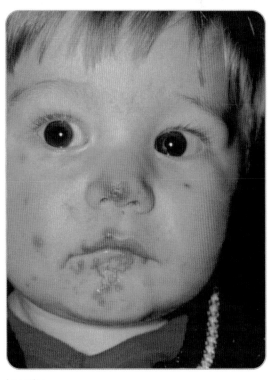

Impetigo

37

The area may appear red and a pustule may be present. Pseudo folliculitis is often referred to as 'razor bumps', and resembles folliculitis without the pus.

Impetigo

A superficial contagious inflammatory disease caused by streptococcal and staphylococcal bacteria. It is commonly seen on the face and around the ears, and features include weeping blisters which dry to form honey-coloured crusts. Bacteria are easily transmitted by dirty fingernails and towels.

Stye

Acute inflammation of a gland at the base of an eyelash, caused by bacterial infection. The gland becomes hard and tender and a pus-filled cyst develops at the centre.

Viral infections of the skin

Herpes simplex (cold sores)

Normally found on the face and around the lips, herpes simplex begins as an itching sensation, followed by erythema and a group of small blisters which then weep and form crusts.

Herpes zoster (shingles)

Painful infection along the sensory nerves caused by the chicken pox virus. The lesions resemble herpes simplex with erythema and blisters along the lines of the nerves. Areas affected are mostly on the back or upper chest wall. Severe pain may persist at the site of shingles for months or even years after the apparent healing of the skin.

Warts

A wart is a benign growth on the skin caused by infection with the human papilloma virus. Plane warts are smooth in texture with a flat top and are usually found on the face, forehead, back of hands and the front of the knees.

Fungal infections of the skin

Ringworm (tinea corporis)

A fungal infection of the skin, which begins as small red papules that gradually increase in size to form a ring. Varies in severity from mild scaling to inflamed itchy areas on the body.

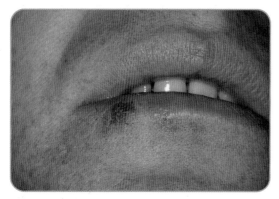

Herpes simplex

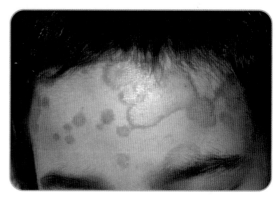

Ringworm

Infestations

Pediculosis (lice)

This is a contagious parasitic infestation where the lice live off blood sucked from the skin. Head lice are frequently seen in young children and if not dealt with quickly, may lead to a secondary infection (impetigo) as a result of scratching. Nits (the eggs), which are pearl-grey or brown, oval structures, may be found on the hair shaft close to the scalp. The scalp may appear red and raw due to scratching.

Body lice are rarely seen. They occur through poor personal hygiene and will live and reproduce in seams and folds of clothing. Lesions may appear as papules, scabs and, in severe cases, pigmented dry, scaly skin. Secondary bacterial infection is often present.

Scabies

A contagious parasitic skin condition, caused by the female mite burrowing into the horny layer of the skin to lay her eggs. The first noticeable symptom of this condition is severe itching which worsens at night; papules, pustules and crusted lesions may also develop.

Common sites for this infestation are the ulnar borders of the hand, palms of the hands and between the fingers and toes. Other sites include the axillary folds, buttocks, breasts in the female and external genitalia in the male.

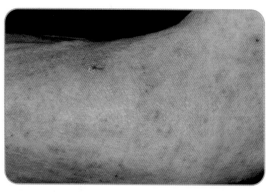

Scabies

Pigmentation disorders

These are not necessarily contraindications to facial treatments, although care does need to be taken with certain pigmentation disorders to avoid stimulation and irritation of the skin, which could further exacerbate an existing condition. The client needs to be advised on how to care for their skin to avoid worsening the disorder and to prevent skin damage.

Albinism

A condition in which there is an inherited absence of pigmentation in the skin, hair and eyes resulting in white hair, pink skin and eyes. The pink colour is produced by underlying blood vessels which are normally masked by pigment. Other clinical signs include poor eyesight and sensitivity to light.

Chloasma

This is a pigmentation disorder which presents with irregular areas of increased pigmentation, usually on the face. It commonly occurs during pregnancy and sometimes through use of the contraceptive pill due to stimulation of melanin by the female hormone oestrogen.

Dermatosis papulosa nigra (DPN)

This is a unique benign skin condition common among black skins. It is characterised by multiple, small, hyperpigmented, asymptomatic papules. It appears as small, dark bumps and most commonly affects the face, neck, chest and back. The cause is uncertain though there is a strong genetic basis for the disorder, and often the lesions can be seen in several members of the same family. The lesions are a type of keratosis that is harmless.

Dermatosis papulosa nigra is not a skin cancer, and it will not turn into a skin cancer. The condition is chronic, with new lesions appearing over time. No treatment is necessary other than for cosmetic concerns. If the lesions are symptomatic (painful, inflamed, itchy, or catch on clothing) they can be treated via a minor surgical procedure.

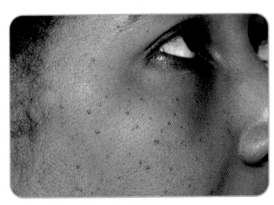

Dermatosis papulosa nigra (DPN)

Lentigo

Also known as 'liver spots'. These are flat dark patches of pigmentation which are found mainly in the elderly on skin exposed to light.

Moles

Moles are also known as a pigmented naevi. They appear as round, smooth lumps on the surface of the skin. They may be flat or raised and vary in size and colour from pink to brown or black. They may have hairs growing out of them.

Naevi

Naevus

A mass of dilated capillaries. May be pigmented as in a birthmark, or vascular as in a portwine stain.

Portwine stain

Also known as a 'deep capillary naevus'. Present at birth, varying in colour from pale pink to deep purple, it has an irregular shape, but is not raised above the skin's surface. Usually found on the face, but may also appear on other areas of the body.

Spider naevi

A collection of dilated capillaries which radiate from a central papule. Often appear during pregnancy or as the result of 'picking a spot'.

Vitiligo (leucoderma)

Areas of the skin lacking pigmentation due to the basal cell layer of the epidermis no longer producing melanin. The cause is unknown.

Hypertrophic disorders

A hypertrophy is an abnormal growth; many are benign or harmless.

Hyperkeratosis

Hyperkeratosis is a rare skin disorder in which there is a gross thickening of the skin due to a mass of keratinocytes that build up to a horny overgrowth of skin cells.

> Note Hyperkeratosis is a common problem for black skins because they desquamate dead skin cells more readily. The accumulation of dead skin cells can give an ashen grey look to black skins. Care needs to be taken to avoid exfoliating too harshly to avoid irritation and sensitivity.

Skin tag

Small growths of fibrous tissue, which stand up from the skin, frequently found on the neck, under the arms and around the breasts. They may be flesh coloured and sometimes are pigmented (black or brown).

> Note Skin tags may be surgically removed or may be cauterised by a qualified electrologist with advanced training. They are not contraindicated to skincare treatment, although care should be taken to avoid catching them and causing any discomfort.

Skin cancers

> Note Any client with an abnormal growth, undiagnosed lump or bump on the skin should be referred to a medical practitioner.

Basal cell carcinoma

A common form of skin cancer that originates in the basal cell layer of the epidermis. Often found on the face and other sun-exposed areas (especially in fair-skinned people). The most common type of basal cell carcinoma is a pearl-like bump, which may be pink or slightly flesh coloured, often with small capillaries running through it. Superficial basal cell carcinomas appear red, flat and scaly and may be misdiagnosed as other conditions, such as eczema.

Basal cell carcinomas rarely spread to other tissues or organs, and although not life threatening they can produce unpleasant scarring if not detected early.

Squamous cell carcinoma

This is a malignant tumour which arises from the prickle cell layer of the epidermis. It is hard and warty and eventually develops a 'heaped-up, cauliflower appearance'. Usually seen in elderly people, it is caused by cumulative sun exposure and occurs more frequently in severely sun-damaged skins.

Unlike basal cell carcinomas, squamous cell carcinomas can spread to other organs, or deeply within the skin. Fortunately 90 per cent of squamous cell carcinomas are detected and removed before they spread.

41

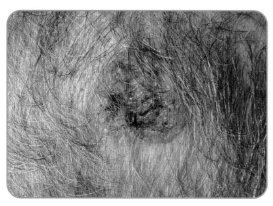

Squamous cell carcinoma

Malignant melanoma

A malignant melanoma is a deeply pigmented mole which is life threatening if it is not

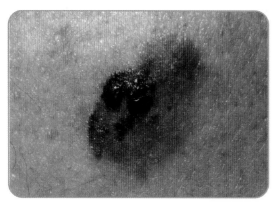

Malignant melanoma

recognised and treated promptly. Its main characteristic is a blue-black nodule which increases in size, shape and colour and is most commonly found on the head, neck and trunk. Overexposure to strong sunlight is a major cause and its incidence is increased in young people with fair skins.

Melanomas can occur in an existing mole or they may arise from normal skin. As they spread very quickly early detection is essential.

It is important to be aware of the typical characteristics of skin cancer:

- An open sore of any size that bleeds, oozes, or crusts and remains open for three or more weeks.
- A persistent non-healing sore.
- A reddish patch or irritated area that doesn't go away, and fails to respond to moisturisers or treatment creams.
- A smooth growth with a distinct rolled border and an indented centre.
- A shiny bump or nodule with a smooth surface that can be pink, red, white, black, brown or purple in colour.
- A white patch of skin that has a smooth, scar-like texture. The area of white stands out from the surrounding skin and can appear clear and taut.

The ABCD of identifying skin cancer:

Asymmetry	One area of the suspected blemish is unlike the other.
Border	An irregular, scalloped edge around the suspected lesion.
Colour	Colour varies from one area to another, and may appear with shades of tan, brown, black, white, red or blue.
Diameter	The area is generally larger than 6 mm.

FAQs: Skin conditions

I have a client who appears to have a form of acne which is very inflamed and is not responding favourably to facial treatments. What advice can you give?

If your client's skin condition is inflamed then advise him to see a GP, who will usually refer him to a dermatologist. Depending on the condition, the GP may prescribe medication (usually a form of antibiotic) to help clear the infection in the follicle that is causing the inflammation. The dermatologist may then recommend a suitable form of treatment or product. Remember that some forms of acne can be helped both medically and aesthetically. Once your client has received the correct medical treatment, he can return to the salon for facial treatments.

When is it advisable to consult a dermatologist regarding skin cancer risk?

It is advisable for clients who have had excessive sun exposure, fair-skinned clients or those with a family history of skin cancer to have annual consultations with a dermatologist. It is also important for any client who has a lot of moles or a history of blistering or severe sunburn reactions to be checked out thoroughly. An important consideration to bear in mind is that it can actually take between 10 and 20 years following a severe sunburn episode for changes to become evident in the skin.

Why are pigmentation problems so difficult to treat? Do any products really help to lighten areas of pigmented skin?

Pigmentation problems are typically harder to treat as the factors that cause them are beyond a therapist's control. The primary cause of pigmentation is sun exposure, however there are other elements such as hormones and genetic skin type. There are skin lightening products on the market such as AHAs and other exfoliating agents which may help, but all products should be used with care to avoid overstimulation and irritation, otherwise the pigmentation may worsen. It is important to explain to clients that it may take months of treatment (salon and homecare) before a change may be seen. It is important to advise the client to avoid sun exposure.

casestudy: rosacea

Debra, 44, had had perfect skin all her life. In her consultation she complained that her skin had suddenly become very sensitive and was reacting to everything she was using. Upon examination under a good light, her skin appeared very red, her cheeks were flushed and although her skin appeared very dry and flaky in places, at the same time there were distinctive red lumps (similar to a breakout) under the skin, which Debra said were very painful. Debra seemed to be showing signs of the skin condition rosacea, but to be sure she received the correct diagnosis and treatment I advised her to seek a dermatologist's advice.

In the meantime, as redness, irritation and skin sensitivity are part of the suspected condition, I advised Debra to examine the products she was currently using and to refrain from using anything stimulating (such as an exfoliant) to avoid exacerbating the condition.

Shortly after the initial consultation Debra returned, with a diagnosis of rosacea from her dermatologist. She was prescribed a topical (antibiotic) gel to help treat the spots under the skin.

We discussed the products she had been using at home and since discontinuing the use of her toner (which happened to contain some AHAs) she had noticed a lessening in the stinging sensation she often experienced following its use. For her initial facial treatment I carried out a basic deep cleansing facial (avoiding massage) using a gentle cleanser, a soothing toner and a gentle, hydrating mask to help decrease the inflammation. The skin responded well to treatment and appeared calm and hydrated afterwards.

As part of Debra's aftercare, I advised her to try to avoid anything which might trigger the flushing such as hot, spicy foods, alcohol, caffeine, hot drinks, stress, strenuous exercise, extremes of temperature, steam from cooking and hot baths or showers. I also advised the use of mild products designed for rosacea or hypersensitivity at home.

A month later Debra returned for her next treatment and having noticed a reduction in the redness, we also included a gentle massage. After three months there was a noticeable reduction in the lumps under the skin and a distinct reduction in redness and sensitivity.

Debra continues to visit the salon for monthly facials, and feels happier and less self-conscious now that her skin condition is under control. Her skin condition is monitored by yearly check ups with her dermatologist.

skin types and conditions

It is essential for the facial therapist to have a good working knowledge of skin types and conditions. Linking skin structure to function will enable the therapist to carry out an effective analysis in order to correctly determine a suitable treatment plan, which will incorporate salon applications, product choice, homecare routine and aftercare advice.

When the skin is in perfect harmony, it appears glowing, beautiful and healthy. If the skin is not in harmony, it will develop problems such as dryness, dehydration, bacterial infection, signs of premature ageing, to name but a few. Every skin will present a combination of types and conditions and before carrying out a skin analysis it is important to know what to look for to guarantee accuracy.

Skin types and their characteristics

The classifications of skin types are determined by genetics and ethnicity. The DNA carried in chromosomes is the factor that programs and influences skin characteristics such as follicle size, skin thickness, circulation and nerve endings.

The primary factors in determining skin types are:

- The level of lipid (fat) secretions that are produced between the skin cells (this determines how well the skin retains moisture).
- The amount of secretion produced by the sebaceous glands.

Skin types are generally broadly classified, and they are often streamlined in the skincare industry to allow clearer marketing of product lines. Skin is generally classified into five main types:

- Normal.
- Dry.
- Oily.
- Combination.
- Sensitive.

Normal skin

Few clients will have normal skin, as this skin type is very rare indeed. Normal skin has a good oil and water balance. The best example of normal skin is in children from birth up until puberty. When questioned the client will usually report that they have very few problems with their skin.

> Note The aim in treating normal skin is to maintain the skin's balance and protect it from damage.

Dry skin

A dry skin is so called because it is either lacking in sebum or moisture, or both. It develops as a result of underactivity of the sebaceous glands. The skin's natural oil, sebum, lubricates the corneum layer and in the absence of this oily coating the dead cells start to curl up and flake. The sebum coating also helps to prevent moisture loss through evaporation, and for this reason dry skin has difficulty retaining inner moisture.

Although dry skin is hereditary, it can also develop as a result of the ageing process. When questioned the client will usually report that their skin feels tight and dry. They may also complain of sensitivity and premature ageing.

> Note The primary aim in treating dry skin is to help to balance the moisture and oil of the skin, soften its texture, and hydrate and moisturise. Dry skin also needs a lot of sun protection.

Oily skin

Oily skin is hereditary, and develops due to an overproduction of sebum from the sebaceous glands. There is always a tendency for clients to overtreat their skin if it is oily; however, this can compound the problem as excessive stimulation results in stripping and irritating the skin, making it become dry and unbalanced. The skin's natural protection mechanism will then respond by producing more oil.

When questioned the client will usually report that their skin develops a 'shine' during the course of a day and make-up runs or 'slips', and maybe their foundation changes to a more orange colour. They will probably complain that their skin often feels thick and dirty, due to the accumulation of sebum and dead cells clogging the surface. They will also suffer with blemishes.

> Note The aim in treating an oily skin is to help balance it, bringing the oil secretions under control by thorough cleansing and exfoliation. It is important to protect and moisturise the surface with a water-based hydrating product designed for oily skin.

Combination skin

This is actually the most common skin type. As its name suggests, this skin is a bit of a mixture; typically the T-zone (central area of the face corresponding to the forehead, nose and chin) is oily and the cheeks and neck are dry/normal. Combination skin can therefore be both dry and oily at the same time.

When questioned the client will usually report that they have all the problems of an oily skin in the T-zone but dryness and tightness on the cheeks, neck and around the eyes. Combination skin presents a dual need to correct the oil and the moisture balance.

Sensitive skin

Whilst sensitivity is a condition that may affect any skin type, sensitive skin is more commonly referred to in its own classification and therefore most product lines now recognise and market products specifically for this skin type.

When questioned the client will probably say their skin reacts easily to external stimuli by becoming red and blotchy, and may feel uncomfortable when touched.

> Note The aim in treating sensitive skin is to soothe and calm the skin, avoiding harsh products and forms of treatment (such as heat) that may cause irritation.

Although all skins may be sensitive at times, due to misuse of products, medication or the environment, clients with genetically determined sensitive skins will have an impaired barrier function and reduced lipid protection, making them more susceptible to allergens and irritants. Caution is therefore essential with this skin type when choosing products and suitable forms of treatment.

Skin type	Hydration	Touch and texture	Other features	Surface appearance	Pores	Elasticity
Normal	Neither too dry, nor too oily	Soft, supple, smooth, neither too thick nor too thin	Slightly warm to touch, good blood supply	Clear, even, free from blemishes	Fine, not noticeable	Good, feels firm
Dry	Dry, often parched	Papery, thin, maybe a little coarse; there may be flaking skin		Often like parchment, dilated capillaries and milia in eye and cheek area, fine lines around eyes	Small and tight	Generally not good
Oily	Oily, shiny, especially in T-zone	Thick and coarse, uneven	Sallow colouring due to excess sebum and dead corneum cell build-up	Usually blocked pores, comedones, papules and pustules; there may be scarring from previous blemishes	Enlarged, due to build-up of sebum	Good, feels firm (oily skin ages least prematurely)
Combination	Dry on cheeks and neck, oily in T-zone	Variable: dry areas rough, oily areas thicker and coarse, patchy	Some sensitivity	Patchy colouring, blemishes in T-zone, perhaps milia and dilated capillaries in drier areas	Variable: as in oily skin in T-zone, fine and small on cheeks	Poor in dry areas, good in oily areas

continued

Skin type	Hydration	Touch and texture	Other features	Surface appearance	Pores	Elasticity
Sensitive	Prone to dry, flaky patches	Warm to touch, thin and translucent	May show high colouring after gentle cleanse, easily irritated by products and external factors	Reddens easily, pink tone, perhaps dilated capillaries	Variables tend to be small and tight	Maybe poor in areas of sensitivity

Ageing of the skin

Like all organs, the skin is affected by the ageing process. In contrast to other organs, changes in the skin become visible over the years. The signs of ageing start to show as early as the end of the second or the beginning of the third decade of a person's life.

The skin's ability to continuously renew itself is affected by ageing. Old skin needs on average twice as long – as much as eight weeks – before it has renewed itself. The natural acidic protective coating changes because the sebaceous and sweat glands no longer exercise their function so efficiently and as the skin becomes drier and thinner it can no longer retain enough moisture and oil.

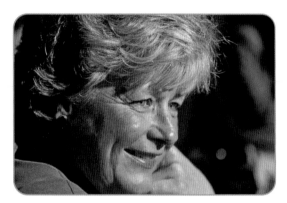

Ageing skin

How age affects the skin

childhood	adolescence	the 20s	the 30s
Smooth, healthy, undamaged.	Sebaceous gland activity, acne, spots, comedones.	Collagen starts to diminish (approx. 1% per year), fine lines, loss of elasticity in skin of upper eyelid.	Sagging due to stretching of the skin and continued reduction in collagen, more fine lines and wrinkles, loss of hydration, moderate decrease in dermal repair.

continued

the 40s	menopause	the 50s	the 60s and beyond
Loss of elasticity more apparent, lines deepen in nasolabial folds, skin sagging at jaw line, forehead wrinkles deepen, noticeable drop in skin hydration levels.	Loss of oestrogen accentuates wrinkles and of elasticity, slowing of ability to synthesise collagen, lipid production affected causing dehydration.	Wrinkles and loss of elasticity in neck more apparent, reduction in supporting fat leads to bonier appearance of face, skin tends to be drier.	Loss of subcutaneous fat, skin thinner, sagging worsens, dilated capillaries often present, uneven pigmentation, age spots, skin tags, low production of sebum and collagen, compromised dermal repair, greater quantity of damaged connective tissue, many wrinkles and deep lines.

Ethnic skin types

The factor that varies in all ethnic skin types is the degree of melanin (the skin's pigment) produced. Although all ethnic skin types have the same number of melanocytes cells, black skins have melanocyte capable of making large amounts of melanin.

White skin

There are relatively small amounts of melanin present in white skins which are of British, Scandinavian, European, North American, South Australian, Canadian, and New Zealand origin. There are those skins which are pale and translucent, often accompanied by freckles and red, blonde or mousy hair. Pale skin is at risk from sunburn, ageing and the formation of skin cancer because of the reduced protection due to the lack of melanin. Pale skins may be unable to develop a tan and may be prone to dehydration and irritation.

Some white skins are far less sensitive, and whilst being pale in the winter may establish a

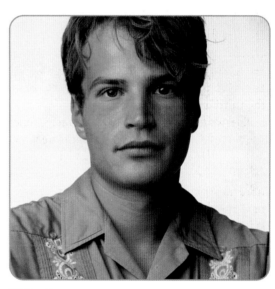
White skin

golden tan easily without burning. Some skins may appear pinkish while others have a sallow tone.

White skins age faster than black skins and it is important, therefore, to start protecting the skin from ultraviolet radiation as early as possible.

49

Oriental/light Asian

This skin type is a creamy colour with a tendency to yellow and olive tones and is of Chinese, Japanese or Middle East origin. There is more melanin present in this skin type. Oriental skin rarely shows blemishes and defies normal signs of ageing. Scars are more likely to occur and hyperpigment, causing unevenness, troughs, pits and hollows on the skin's surface.

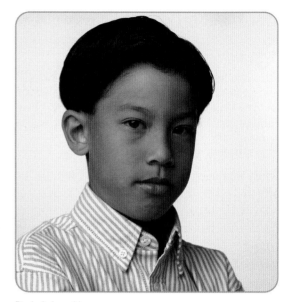

Dark Asian skin

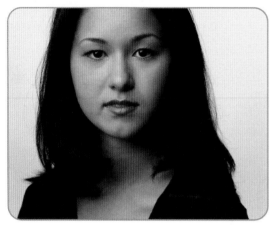

Oriental/light Asian skin

Dark Asian skin

This is a very dark skin colour, of Pakistani, Indian, Sri Lankan, or Malaysian origin, which is deeply pigmented with melanin. Dark Asian skin is smooth and supple with minimal signs of ageing. Sweat glands are larger and more numerous in this skin type which gives a sheen to the skin that is often mistaken for oiliness. As this skin type is deeply pigmented it does not reveal the blood capillaries.

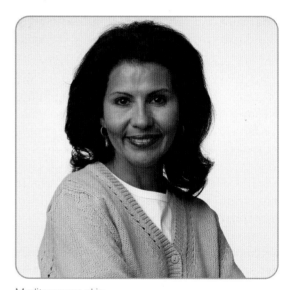

Mediterranean skin

Mediterranean-type skin

This skin type, of Italian, Spanish, Greek, Portuguese, Yugoslavian or South and Central American origin, presents as sallow with some reddish pigment and tans easily and deeply without burning. There is a good degree of melanin present which obscures the colour of the blood vessels. Mediterranean-type skin tends to have a generous coating of sebum and is therefore oily.

Afro-Caribbean/black skin

Black skins, of West Indian or African origin, have a higher degree of sebum as sebaceous glands are larger, more numerous and closer to the skin's surface with open pores. As black skin is thicker than white skins it is prone to congestion and comedones. This skin type is tough, desquamates easily, forms keloid scars when damaged and is also more likely to be affected by several different types of disfiguring bumps. Dermatosis papulosa nigra (DPN) is a benign cutaneous condition that is common among black skins (see Chapter 3, page 40).

> Note Keloid scars are thick and lumpy and often extend beyond the borders of the wound.

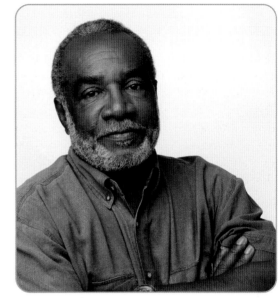

Afro-Caribbean skin

Black skin generally ages at a much slower rate than white skin, mainly due to the extra protection from sun damage afforded by the melanin. A disadvantage to having more melanin is that it makes the skin more 'reactive'. This means that almost any stimulus – a rash, scratch or inflammation – may trigger the production of excess melanin, resulting in dark marks or patches on the skin. This is known as post-inflammatory hyperpigmentation.

Less commonly, some black skins develop a decrease in melanin, or post-inflammatory hypopigmentation in response to skin trauma. In either case the light or dark areas may be disfiguring and may take months or years to fade.

The increased thickness of the horny layer of the skin in black skins can cause dehydration which leads to increased skin shedding. This can create a grey 'ashen' effect as the loose cells build up on the skin.

Mixed skin

Clients with a mixed skin will usually have a combination of characteristics of all of the above skin types. The shades of colour and characteristics will vary greatly depending on the mix.

Fitzpatrick skin types

Developed by a dermatologist, Dr Thomas Fitzpatrick, the Fitzpatrick Scale is a method of analysing the skin's tolerance to sun exposure, and can be a valuable gauge in assessing how reactive a skin may be to advanced skincare methods such as chemical peels, laser treatment and microdermabrasion.

Whilst Fitzpatrick skin types I–III tend to be more reactive to topical substances and environmental factors, pigmentation problems are more likely to affect skin types IV–VI (as the skin is more reactive to stimulation and injuries).

Fitzpatrick skin type	Appearance	Skin's reaction to sun exposure
Type I	Very fair, blonde or red hair Light coloured eyes Freckles are common	Always burns, never tans
Type II	Fair skinned Blonde or red hair Blue, green or hazel eyes	Burns easily, tans with difficulty
Type III	Very common skin type; fair Eye and hair colour varies	Sometimes burns, gradually tans
Type IV	Moderately pigmented skin	Rarely burns, always tans
Type V	Medium to heavy pigmentation	Very rarely burns, tans easily
Type VI	Black skin, deeply pigmented	Least sensitive, tans well

Skin conditions

Skin conditions develop over a period of time and can apply to all skin types. Common examples which may be encountered during a facial treatment include acne, comedones, blocked/enlarged pores, papules, pustules, dehydration, milia, wrinkles, sun damage, sensitivity, dehydration, poor elasticity and pigmentation problems.

Causes of skin conditions may be internal or external. Some conditions may be significantly improved by regular facial treatment, use of the correct products and clients following the correct advice. It is important for the therapist to be able to recognise them and be able to offer or recommend a suitable method of treatment.

Acne

Acne normally affects adolescents between the ages of 14 and 20 and has normally regressed by the age of 25. A form of adult acne may also occur later in life due to hormonal or other factors. See Chapter 3, pages 31–3 for more information on acne.

Blocked pores

When sebum begins to build up in a pore, the pore will appear enlarged and sebaceous matter inside will be evident. The excess sebum needs to be released to prevent further build-up within the pore.

Enlarged pores

Larger pores are due to excess oil and debris trapped in the hair follicles, or expansion due to loss of elasticity.

Comedone

A blocked follicle (see Chapter 3, page 33 for information on comedones).

Dehydration

Water intake is necessary for the healthy functioning of the body and skin's cells. Dehydration means that there is a lack of moisture in the intercellular system of the skin. Key indicators of dehydration are visible fine lines and a feeling of tightness on the skin.

Dehydration can affect any skin type, even an oily skin. Dehydration in oily skin is usually a result of using products that are too harsh which have stripped the skin of its protective coating of sebum. Many skin types can suffer from temporary dehydration, such as that caused through illness, medication, over-exposure to the elements (cold, wind, and heat), central heating and dehydrating drinks such as caffeine and alcohol.

As well as a dehydrated skin presenting a parched, dry looking, rough surface, it will also tend to soak up any product applied very quickly.

Dilated capillaries

The technical term for dilated capillaries is telangiectasis (often called couperose). This condition presents as diffused areas of redness on the cheeks, nose and neck, occurring primarily as a result of poor elasticity in the capillary wall. It is caused by sun exposure, smoking, alcohol, or poor health, in fact any factor which puts stress on the capillaries.

Lines and wrinkles

Once the underlying structure of the skin has become damaged and the skin starts to lose its elasticity, exaggerated lines and wrinkles start to form on the face and neck. These may be formed as a result of the normal ageing process, but often are prematurely formed due to sun and environmental damage.

The fine lines around the eye area, known as 'crows feet', appear with age and are precipitated by squinting and exposure to ultraviolet light (not wearing adequate protection for the eyes). They may also be aggravated by rough handling of the skin when removing cosmetics.

Milia

White pearly lumps that appear under the skin (see Chapter 3, page 33 for more information on milia).

Pigmentation problems

Pigmentation may be associated with a client's ethnic skin type, or may be caused by environmental or other factors. Pigmentation problems may result from the uneven distribution of melanin over the skin's surface, either due to an accumulation of pigment, or because of uneven production by the melanocytes. The melanocyte cells are located in the basal cell layer of the epidermis, and they surround a large number of regular skin cells (keratinocytes).

Melanin production varies from individual to individual, and is greater in those with darker skins. Melanin acts as a filter to help protect the skin against the harmful effects of the sun's radiation. Any surface irritation of the skin (including exposure to the sun) is capable of increasing melanin production.

Hyperpigmentation

This is an excess of skin pigment, resulting in brown discoloration/darkening of the skin. The overproduction of pigment results when the melanocytes produce a greater amount of melanin in a given area of the skin and/or when the melanin is not properly absorbed by the keratinocytes.

Hyperpigmentation is usually caused by exposure to the sun or environmental damage, although a type of hyperpigmentation may occur during pregnancy (chloasma). Hyperpigmentation may also result from injuries, rashes or chemical irritation, and is especially common in darker skins.

Hypopigmentation

This condition presents as white, colourless areas resulting from less than normal melanin production, or the absence of pigmentation. It may be due to long-term sun exposure or irritation, which causes a dysfunction in the melanocytes.

Poor elasticity

Poor elasticity, or elastosis, resulting in sagging or loose skin is a sign of ageing or damage from the sun.

Puffiness/dark circles

Puffiness and dark circles around the eyes are usually a sign of fatigue, which may be related to lifestyle. They may also indicate poor elimination of waste (impaired lymphatic drainage) which causes a build-up of toxins in the system, or a poor diet (with too much sugar, starch or salt). However, some ethnic skin types present with a natural darkness around the eyes due to the distribution of pigment in the skin.

Sensitivity

Sensitivity is a condition that may affect any skin type, and should not be confused with genetically predisposed sensitive skin. Sensitivity will usually manifest itself as redness, itching or burning. Because the chemical composition of each person's skin varies, one client may react sensitively to an ingredient, while another may not.

> Note It is important to note that an ingredient may not be sensitising as a rule, but a client's skin may be sensitive to that particular ingredient. An ingredient can only be deemed sensitising if most clients react to it with sensitivity.

Sensitivity and allergies may occur due to exposure to specific product ingredients, misuse of products, medication, diet, or factors such as hot and cold weather or the wind. Major ingredients that can cause sensitivity are those found in fragrances, preservatives and some chemical sunscreens.

Sun damage/photoageing

The main cause of premature ageing is sun damage (photoageing) and is directly related to the effects of prolonged or excessive sun exposure.

Sunlight is made up of different wavelengths of light, and the earth's atmosphere allows visible light, ultraviolet A (UVA) and ultraviolet B (UVB) through. This light causes premature

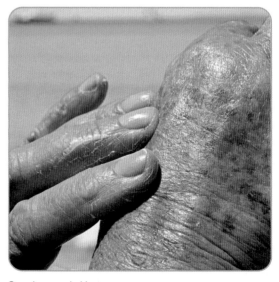

Sun-damaged skin

ageing by directly breaking down the skin's support structures, namely collagen and elastin. It also damages the enzymes that protect collagen from breakdown.

Sun-damaged skins will present with much deeper lines and wrinkles than undamaged skin of the same age. Lines and wrinkles will also be present in areas other than those with normal expression lines. The texture will tend to be rougher, thicker and dehydrated. There may be areas of diffuse redness (due to more prominent blood vessels) and uneven pigmentation. The skin will lack elasticity due to the collagen and elastin breakdown.

Factors affecting the skin

There are many factors, both external and internal, which affect a client's skin.

Internal factors affecting the skin

Age

The process of ageing naturally affects the skin, as cell regeneration starts to decrease with age (see the chart on page 57 for information on the effects of ageing).

Free radicals

These also contribute to skin ageing. Free radicals are parts of molecules (e.g. oxygen molecules) that are found in the body. As a result of external factors, like ultraviolet radiation, nicotine or unhealthy food, the free radicals become prone to react and are constantly looking for other chemical substances to bond with. Hence, they attack the collagen fibres, cellular membrane and lipid layer of the skin. Free radicals change the inherited properties stored in the cell nucleus, so that the quality of newly formed skin cells deteriorates.

The body protects itself against these aggressors through antioxidant enzyme systems (antioxidants). But from the age of 20 onwards, these natural defence mechanisms gradually decline and the skin can no longer defend itself. Making up for the hormone and antioxidant deficiencies caused by ageing by supplying the body with hormone and vitamin supplements is one of the basic ideas of modern anti-ageing therapy.

Stress and lifestyle

When the body is subjected to regular stress and tension it can cause sensitivity and allergies in the skin as well as encourage the formation of lines around the eyes and the mouth.

Hormones

The natural glandular changes of the body have an effect on the condition of the skin. During puberty, the sex hormones stimulate the sebaceous glands, which may cause imbalance in the skin.

At the onset of menstruation the skin may erupt due to the adjustment of hormones levels. During pregnancy, pigmentation changes may occur, but usually disappear at delivery. During the menopause the activity of the sebaceous glands is reduced and the skin becomes drier.

Smoking

The effects of smoking have been linked to premature ageing and wrinkling of the skin. Nicotine weakens the blood vessels supplying blood to the tissues, depriving the tissues of essential oxygen, and therefore the skin may appear dull and grey in colour. Smoking affects the skin's cells and destroys vitamins B and C which are important for healthy skin.

Smoking also dulls the skin by polluting the pores and increases the formation of lines around the eyes and the mouth.

Medication

Medication can affect the skin by causing dehydration, or sensitivity and/or allergies.

Skin enhancing vitamins

A	Helps repair body tissues, prevents dryness and ageing.
B	Improves circulation and skin colour; essential to cellular oxidation.
C	Essential for healing, maintains levels of collagen.
E	Heals damaged tissues and structural damage to skin.

Water consumption

The skin is approximately 70 per cent water. Drinking an adequate amount of water (approximately 6–8 glasses per day) aids the digestive system and helps prevent a build-up of toxicity in the skin's tissues.

Alcohol

Alcohol has a dehydrating effect on the skin by drawing essential water from the tissues. Excess consumption causes the blood vessels in the skin to dilate, resulting in a flushed appearance.

Exercise

Regular exercise promotes good circulation, increased oxygen intake and blood flow to the skin.

Sleep

Sleep is essential to physical and emotional well-being and is one of the most effective regenerators for the skin.

Diet

A healthy body is needed for a healthy skin. The skin can be thought of as a barometer of the body's general health.

External factors affecting the skin

Photoageing

Although sun damage (see page 53) is the one of the most significant factors in photoageing of the skin, it is important to note that tanning machines/sunbeds can also cause accelerated ageing of the skin due to the fact that they produce large quantities of long wave ultraviolet light (UVA). Overexposure may lead to the same risks as overexposure to natural sunlight, i.e. sagging and wrinkling and an increased risk of some skin cancers.

Environmental exposure

Exposure to adverse weather conditions (such as wind, rain, cold, heat and sudden changes in temperature), pollutants, or poor air quality can affect the condition of the skin, often resulting in dryness and dehydration.

Occupation

The client's occupation could be a factor affecting their skin condition, for example, if they work in a hot or humid environment, or in dusty and dirty conditions.

Poor care

Lack of, or incorrect, skincare can be a major factor affecting the skin's condition. The use of products that are too aggressive can strip the skin and effectively damage the barrier function of the skin. The correct use of sunscreens can provide the best protection against premature ageing.

> **Note** It is essential to advise clients who work outdoors or participate in outdoor activities (sailing, gardening) to take adequate precautions to avoid a 'weather-beaten' skin.

FAQs: Skin types and conditions

At what age should you start to think about looking after your skin?

Skin is often beautifully smooth and normal, and usually at its most healthy and undamaged state during childhood but it is never too early to learn about skincare. The care of the skin during childhood is almost entirely in the hands of the parents or carers and it is vital they protect children's skins against the damaging effects of the sun to prevent the development of skin cancer in later years. Teaching good skincare habits at a young age will help maintain a healthy skin for a lifetime.

I have heard that essential fatty acids are important to the health of the skin. Why is this?

Essential fatty acids, found in vegetable oils, nuts and cereals, are a vital part of the daily diet as they cannot be manufactured by the body. They are important to the health of the skin as they form a key part of the skin's barrier by maintaining an adequate lipid (fat) supply in the epidermis, as well as controlling the speed at which healthy cells are produced.

Does dry skin cause wrinkles?

Most of the lines and wrinkles that you see are caused by sun damage and/or smoking, and to a lesser extent by facial expressions such as smiling and frowning. The reason most people believe that dry skin causes wrinkles is that if the skin is very dehydrated it can seem more wrinkled. As you age, the skin produces less sebum, which can make wrinkling more apparent.

Is there anything that can be done to minimise the effects of sun damage from the past?

It is never too later to start protecting the skin from the sun. It is the cumulative effects that cause the damage, so by avoiding exposure you could halt some of its progress and there is some evidence that you can still benefit from reducing sun exposure in later life. With clients who have what's called actinic keratoses (pre-cancerous skin lesions) it has been noted that limiting their sun exposure actually reduces these lesions, even at a relatively late stage. Because non-melanoma forms of skin cancer are linked with cumulative sun exposure that's a very good reason for clients to be advised to alter their sun exposure habits.

57

casestudy: sun damage

Upon consultation, the outer layer of 49-year-old Carol's skin appeared wrinkled, thickened, and yellowy in colour. By her own admission, Carol had not used adequate sun protection for her skin and, like many clients, did not realise that signs of past sun damage do not become evident until around the 40s to 50s.

Carol's skin felt quite leathery to the touch with a significant degree of elastosis (loss of elasticity) due to the destruction of the collagen and elastin in the dermis. Her skin also felt very dehydrated, and when questioned about her skincare regime at home, Carol reported that as her skin had been oily up until her 40s she had never used a moisturiser as she felt it would made her skin more shiny.

I suggested we commenced with a course of four superficial mild alpha hydroxy acid skin peels (25 per cent strength) to help to normalise the over-thickened skin (hyperkeratinisation) and to help promote a healthy glow to reduce the visible signs of ageing. Carol was advised to avoid any changes to her skincare regime for one week prior to treatment (i.e. avoid sunbathing, exfoliation, waxing and use of new products). Each treatment, 30 minutes in duration (carried out at twice monthly intervals), commenced with the use of a cleanser to help degrease and remove the skin's protective oil in order to allow a more uniform penetration of the glycolic acid into the skin.

After treatment the skin appeared pink, but there was no discomfort, only a mild stinging sensation when the solution was applied. For aftercare Carol was advised to cleanse her skin with a gentle cleanser, to keep the skin hydrated by moisturising twice daily and avoid sun exposure, as well as applying a sunscreen. She was also advised to avoid exfoliating her skin and to avoid picking or peeling away any scales of dead skin.

After each treatment Carol's skin appeared smoother, softer and less thickened, brighter and with a healthier colour. The most significant changes were noted after about six weeks, by which time Carol was so pleased with the renewed appearance of her skin that she continued to attend the salon for rejuvenating facials with the use of anti-ageing AHA products at home. Carol was also advised to have a maintenance peel once every couple of months, in between her regular facials at the salon.

client consultation and skin analysis

Being able to carry out a thorough analysis of the skin is an essential first step to providing a professional skincare service. Every client's skin will be different and will present different challenges. Clients rely on professional advice to help improve the appearance of their skin, whether it is dealing with blemishes and breakout or the signs of ageing. A consultation and skin analysis is also an effective marketing opportunity to recommend the correct facial products and treatments, and to raise client awareness of the benefits of professional skincare.

> Note The very essence of client assessment and skin analysis is in communication and observation.

Client consultation

A thorough client consultation is essential in order to gather the relevant information relating to the client's skin condition.

The consultation is an opportunity to:

- Identify any contraindications or conditions that may prevent or restrict treatment.
- Determine the need for any special care (such as sensitive skin, rosacea or acne).
- Find out what the client wants from the treatment.
- Determine what the client's skin needs from the treatment.
- Explain the proposed form of treatment and agree a treatment plan.
- Answer the client's questions.
- Promote the sale of products and facial services that will benefit the client's skin.

Accurate record keeping is essential in helping evaluate and present information on the client's skin type and current condition (the skin analysis). Asking the client questions relating to their health, lifestyle and current skin routine will provide information on the probable causes of their skin problems.

Client records will also contain details of treatments carried out, products used and results, as well as the recommended homecare programme.

Contraindications to facials

As facials are designed to improve the condition of the skin, they should never be applied where there is infection, damage, in the case of a client with a serious medical condition, or where there is a risk of an adverse reaction. Therapists need to be able to recognise and respond in a professional manner to contraindications as failure to do so may result in cross-infection, interfering with the healing process or worsening the existing condition.

There are three main categories of contraindications to facials:

1 Those totally contraindicated; where treatment should not be given.

2 Those requiring medical referral.

3 Those restricting treatment.

Total contraindications

a) Any form of infection or disease, e.g.

- An infectious skin condition such as impetigo, herpes simplex, tinea/ringworm, or a client suffering from an acute infectious disease such as flu.
- An eye infection such as conjunctivitis or a stye.
- Fever/elevated temperature, indicating possible infections and illness.
- Illness, such as diarrhoea or vomiting.

b) A client under the influence of recreational drugs or alcohol.

c) Any known allergies/allergic reactions where there is a risk of an adverse reaction.

> Note Information from the client is needed to establish the nature of any allergy and its effects. If a client has a known allergy to a certain ingredient or product, then the facial treatment may be provided by avoiding contact with known allergens.

Contraindications that may require medical referral

Circulatory disorders

Such as:

- Heart conditions.
- Medical oedema (general accumulation of fluid due to kidney or heart disease).
- Thrombosis.
- Phlebitis.
- High or low blood pressure.

> Note Clients presenting with high blood pressure are likely to have redness of the face and facial swelling. If the client is suitable for treatment, it is important to avoid heat and other stimulants.

Nervous system disorders

Such as:

- Epilepsy.
- Multiple sclerosis.
- Parkinson's disease.
- Motor neurone disease.
- Pinched/trapped nerve.
- Inflamed nerves (Bell's Palsy).
- Slipped disc.

- Spastic conditions.
- Nervous/psychotic conditions.

Musculoskeletal disorders

Such as:

- Osteoporosis.
- Acute arthritis (osteo or rheumatoid).
- Acute rheumatism.
- Postural deformities.
- Whiplash/conditions affecting the neck.
- Cervical spondylitis (inflammation of the synovial joints of the cervical vertebrae, causing pain and stiffness).

Severe skin conditions

Such as:

- Severe acne (Grade III or IV).
- Severe eczema, dermatitis or psoriasis.

Skin cancer

Or evidence of suspected malignant tumours.

Diabetes

Some clients with diabetes may have skin that presents as thin and papery, and therefore their skin condition may be considered unstable and they may be unable to give feedback fully regarding pressure. Caution should be exercised as some diabetic clients may have acute complications such as hypoglycaemia, resulting in dizziness, weakness, pallor, rapid heartbeat and excessive sweating.

Asthma

As asthma is a chronic inflammatory disease of the lungs, it affects a client's breathing. It is important to always obtain a detailed history during the consultation stage, specifically on the triggers that cause an attack. If the client has a history of allergies, ensure they are not allergic to any preparations or substances you may be proposing to use. Position the clients according to their individual comfort, usually in a semi-reclined position in order to ensure that breathing is not impaired. It is usually advisable to avoid the use of steam.

Undiagnosed pain, lumps or swellings

These need to be investigated before any treatment is offered.

Prescribed medication

Some forms of medication may cause the skin to react more readily to any form of stimulation and the skin may become more sensitive to treatment as a result.

Contraindications restricting treatment

- Recent scar tissue.
- Recent surgery.
- Recent fractures or soft tissue injuries.
- Hormonal implants.
- Headache/migraine.
- Botox (avoid facial treatment for 1 week following treatment to ensure no migration of Botox occurs).
- Dermal fillers (avoid the treated area for 2 weeks following treatment due to possible tenderness and swollen tissues).
- Sunburn.
- Hypersensitive skins.
- Areas of inflammation, soreness, irritation, cuts, abrasions or bruising.

The facial consultation

The facial consultation form reflects the consultation process itself:

✑ The first part is devoted to the initial consultation and contraindication check.

✑ The second part is the skin analysis.

✑ The third part is the treatment and product records.

Facial consultation form

Personal Information

Client's name _____   Reference number _____

Address

_____

_____

Contact telephone numbers:

Home _____   Work _____   Mobile _____

Date of birth _____   Occupation _____

Medical Information

Contraindications checklist

Do you have/are you currently affected by any of the following? (please circle and give details below)

Any form of infection or disease?

Circulatory disorder? heart condition / thrombosis / phlebitis / high or low blood pressure / medical oedema / other (please state below)

Nervous system disorder? epilepsy / multiple sclerosis / Parkinson's disease / motor neurone disease / pinched / trapped nerve / inflamed nerves (Bell's Palsy) / slipped disc / spastic conditions nervous / psychotic conditions / other (please state below)

Skeletal system disorder? osteoporosis / osteoarthritis / rheumatoid arthritis / postural deformities / whiplash / conditions affecting the neck / cervical spondylitis / other (please state below)

Skin disorder? acne / psoriasis / eczema / skin cancer / other (please state below)

Any skin infections? tinea (fungal infections) / impetigo / boils / scabies / herpes (please state below)

Any eye infections? conjunctivitis / stye

Diabetes?

Asthma?

Facial consultation form *continued*

Any undiagnosed pain/lumps or swellings?

Recent surgery or operation?

Recent fractures or soft tissue injuries?

Hormonal implants?

Recent scar tissue?

Headache/migraine?

Sunburn?

Hypersensitive skin?

Areas of inflammation, soreness, irritation, cuts, abrasions or bruising?

Have you had any form of cosmetic treatments such as Botox/dermal fillers?

Details of any condition indicated above

_____

_____

Do you have any known allergies to foods, cosmetic or drugs/medication? (please give details below)

_____

_____

Do you have any condition (medical or other) that has not been mentioned above?

_____

Are you currently under a doctor's/dermatologist's care for any skin condition, or other problem? Please give details

_____

_____

Doctor's name _____

Surgery _____

Are you currently taking any medication?

_____

_____

Lifestyle and Diet

Typical daily diet _____

_____

Facial consultation form *continued*

Daily fluid intake _____

Vitamin supplements taken _____

Do you smoke? _____

Are your sleep patterns   good/average/poor?

Are your stress levels   high/average/low?

What do you do to relax and unwind?

_____

Current Skincare Regime

Which of the following products do you currently use?

soap / cleanser / toner / exfoliator / moisturiser / sunscreen / mask / eye cream

Others (please state)

_____

Please state the brand you are currently using, and the regime/routine you follow.

_____

General Information

Is this the first time you have sought professional skincare advice and treatment? Yes/No
(*please give details of previous salon treatment and products used*)

_____

_____

How would you describe your current skin condition?

_____

_____

What are the main concerns you have about your skin?

_____

_____

Client Signature/Agreement

I understand that the information given is completely confidential and is an aid to helping the therapist to give a better service. I do not knowingly suffer from any condition that prevents me from having a facial.

Client's signature _____   **Date** _____

Skin analysis

A skin analysis is carried out after the skin has been cleansed and prior to all other treatments. The skin can only be analysed accurately once all the surface secretions have been removed. Skin analysis is not difficult, it is just a question of being methodical, looking carefully and asking the correct questions.

Skin magnification

An essential factor in skin analysis is the use of a magnifying lamp. A typical magnifying lamp, with a cool fluorescent light bulb, magnifies the face and enables the therapist to analyse the skin accurately.

A Wood's Lamp can be used to illuminate the health of the skin and pigmentation and other skin problems. This lamp has a filtered black light and enables the therapist to carry out a more in-depth skin analysis. The treatment room must be totally dark when using the lamp, which reflects the different shades of colour of a client's skin. Some examples of skin conditions and how they appear under a Wood's Lamp are:

- Thick horny layer = white fluorescence.
- Layer of dead skin cells (horny layer) = white spots.
- Normal healthy skin = blue-white.
- Dehydration = light violet.
- Oily areas/comedones = yellow or sometimes pink.
- Pigmentation problems = brown.

Note Whichever form of magnifier is used, it is important to check the equipment, and ensure all adjustment knobs and fixings are secure before use. Remember to protect a client's eyes from the light by securing some small eye pads on the eyelids.

Always turn the lamp on away from the client before bringing it over the client's face. The bulbs do get hot so care needs to be taken to ensure the bulb does not touch the client's skin and that it is not turned on for too long.

In addition to a good magnifying light, the essential tools needed to carry out an effective skin analysis are:

- The eyes to observe colour, pigmentation, pore size, blemishes, sensitivity, lines and wrinkles in order to assess the client's skin condition.
- The ears for listening to the client's account of their skin problems.
- The hands to assess factors such as temperature, texture, hydration levels, elasticity and thickness of the skin.

When carrying out a skin analysis it is helpful to divide the skin and neck into areas or zones, like on a map. You can then work methodically through each of the numbered areas and note down what you can see on the skin analysis form.

Zone 1 – neck

The neck is often a neglected area. Due to its lack of bony support and small amount of supporting fat, the skin on the neck can be stretched very easily. The neck can quickly show signs of ageing if not looked after, as there are very few sebaceous glands in this area and the skin can become dry and crêpey, particularly if it is not protected from the harmful effects of UV light. Most clients think about protecting their faces from the sun but not their necks.

The neck can quickly lose fat through dieting or illness and this can give an aged appearance. As people age there is also a gradual loss of fat from the neck, causing the platysma muscle to become more evident. As maturity sets in, particularly if the neck skin is dry, horizontal lines (sometimes called necklace lines) can develop and can become quite deep.

Zone 2: chin, jaw and mouth

As the chin is part of the T-zone and contains more active sebaceous glands than other parts of the face it can tend to suffer with blocked pores, comedones, papules and pustules, especially in younger clients. Special attention needs to be paid to the horizontal crease in the chin as this is a prime site for congestion.

As we age, muscles in the lower part of the face lose tone and it is possible for a 'double-chin' and jowls to appear. The lips and mouth also become smaller as the gums shrink, pulling the skin of the lips inward. Many clients lose a definite lipline and vertical lines appear above the upper lip. Smoking greatly encourages these lines to develop. Some hair growth may also develop on the upper lip, particularly as a client ages.

> Note Recommend to clients that they keep their lips well protected at all times. The lips can easily dry out and become badly chapped. As the lips do not contain melanin it is possible for them to burn in the sun and there is actually quite a high incidence of lip cancer.

Zone 3: nose

Like the chin, the nose is part of the T-zone and is abundantly supplied with large sebaceous glands. The nose is often oily and plagued by the formation of blocked pores, comedones, papules and pustules. The sides of the nose are often affected most due to the accumulation of excess sebum here and careful attention must be paid to thorough cleansing and extraction.

The skin on the top of the nose is often very fine as it is stretched tightly over the nasal bone with little supporting tissue. It is easily

damaged through exposure to the elements, rough handling, or harsh products. The capillaries often rupture and remain permanently dilated and visible on the skin's surface – the result is a very red nose which looks worse when the client is warm. The capillaries can also rupture if the client often blows her nose (i.e. a frequent cold or hay fever sufferer) or if an incorrect skincare regime has been carried out.

> Note The nose must always be well protected from the elements by a good moisturiser, but take care that it is not too greasy and heavy for this area.

Zones 4 and 5: cheeks

In youth the skin in this area is usually smooth, firm and plump. As we age the cheeks lose their underlying muscle and fat support and as the moisture content also reduces, a hollow, gaunt appearance can result, especially in people who are quite thin or have suddenly lost a lot of weight very quickly.

As there is a loss of muscle tone in the risorius and zygomatic muscles, which both insert at the corners of the mouth, the characteristic nasolabial lines form (mouth to nose lines). There is not such an abundance of sebaceous glands in the skin over the cheeks so dryness and dehydration can be a problem. Good moisturisation is essential.

On the upper part of the cheekbones, nearer the eyes, the skin is often finer as it stretches over the zygomatic arch and the capillaries rise more closely to the surface. If exposed to the elements or treated harshly it is common to find dilated capillaries here and, if severe, a very red complexion can develop. Milia may also form around this part of the face as the skin is often drier.

Zone 6: eyes

The skin around the eyes and forming the eyelids is extremely thin and must be treated with the greatest of care. There are very few sebaceous glands in the skin around the eyes and there is often a lot of dryness.

As the delicate muscle that surrounds the eye (orbicularis oculi) loses tone, a slackness can be noticed above the upper lid. Fine lines then form at the sides of the eye and are further exacerbated by screwing up the eyes, for instance in bright sunlight and when smoking. Through ageing the skin becomes much thinner and the blood supply is easily visible, showing through as a purplish-blue colour. A division between the point at which the lower eyelid meets the cheek becomes noticeable and a semi-circular depression is left. Some people suffer with dark circles below the eyes, which can be due to insufficient sleep, hereditary factors or ill health.

Puffiness around the eyes is also a common problem, due to insufficient sleep, allergies, sinus congestion or creams that are too heavy and clog the pores. It is important to choose a cream formulated specifically for use around the delicate eye area. As we age it is possible for a permanently puffy appearance to result around the eyes as fat and fluid herniate through the very delicate orbicularis oculi muscle. Milia are often found on this fine, dry skin.

Zone 7: forehead

As part of the T-zone, the forehead can suffer from excess oiliness, blocked pores, comedones, papules and pustules. Some clients wear a heavy fringe which can further exacerbate the problem. The skin stretches tightly over the frontal bone that lies below with very little supporting fat. As the skin ages and tone is lost in the frontalis muscle, horizontal ridges begin to form. Vertical

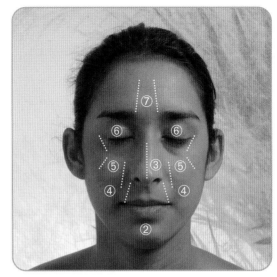

Facial map

ƒ creases between the eyebrows become noticeable as ageing and factors such as eyestrain or frowning contribute to their formation.

Questioning the client

It is important to avoid making a superficial diagnosis when analysing a client's skin, as establishing the correct skin type and condition has implications for the effectiveness of the chosen course of facial treatment. Gather as much information as possible through observation, touch and questioning the client.

It is essential to know about the client's current skincare routine, as inappropriate products for their skin type may be the cause of their current skin condition. Questioning the client will help you make judgements about the skin and conditions present.

Useful questions to ask:

- How does your skin generally feel?
- How would you summarise your main problems?
- Does your skin absorb products easily?

🔖 Does your skin react easily to products/treatments?

🔖 Have you had any problems with your skin in the past (such as acne)?

Note It is essential that a skin analysis is carried out during each facial treatment, as the skin will change and it is the current condition that needs to be treated.

Recording skin analysis findings

When analysing a client's skin it is necessary to take account of each of the following factors.

Important factors in skin analysis

Skin colour	Indicates health and current condition. Bluish coloration may indicate poor circulation. Redness or couperose may arise from vascular and follicular dilation. Pigment plays a major role in the colour of the skin.
Pigmentation	Conditions relating to abnormal melanin production must be noted. Abnormal distribution of melanin may be due to sun damage, injury, irritation, hormones or ethnic skin type.
Skin texture	Relates to the process of cell renewal. A build-up of dead cells can make the skin feel rough.
Thickness	Dry and sensitive skins will tend to feel thinner, oilier skins thicker.
Pore size	Oily skins have open pores, dry and sensitive skins barely visible pores. Loss of elasticity of the follicles (due to acne for instance) can be seen in mature clients with dry skin.
Hydration levels	Signs of dehydration may include a rough, flaky appearance, fine lines and sun damage. Dehydrated skin shows first signs of ageing.
Sebaceous secretions	A good indicator is whether there is any shine to the skin.
Blemishes	Skin blockages: comedones, papules and pustules.
Elasticity	Skin lacking elasticity will tend to feel soft and flaccid, rather than firm and tight, as in a well-toned skin. To test for skin elasticity gently lift the skin between the thumb and forefinger and then release. If the skin snaps back quickly it has good elasticity. If the skin takes any time to snap back it is lacking elasticity.
Muscle tone	Loss of muscle tone may be evident visually (typically around the jaw line) or may be tested manually (see above: elasticity of the skin).
Lines and wrinkles	May be superficial or deep; an indication of how the skin is ageing.
Sensitivity	Gauge how reactive the skin is by gentle touching, and by questioning the client as to intolerance to specific products.
Eyes	Condition of skin around the eyes may indicate a client's lifestyle, or may be due to their ethnic skin type.

Below is an example of the second part of the client's facial record: the Individual Skin Analysis Record.

Individual skin analysis record

Skin colour	pale / medium / tanned / olive / dark / black
Circulation	good / normal / poor
Pigmentation	normal / hyperpigmentation / hypopigmentation
Skin texture	smooth / rough / granular
Thickness of skin	fine / slightly thick / thick and heavy
Pore size	very fine (not visible) / fine (visible) / moderate (more visible) / enlarged
Hydration levels	normal / superficial dehydration / deep dehydration
Secretion levels	normal / low / moderate / high
Blemishes	comedones: (open / closed) / papules / pustules / cysts / scars / milia
Elasticity	firm / mild loss of tone / severe loss of tone
Muscle tone	good / average / poor
Lines and wrinkles	superficial / deep
Sensitivity	normal / reactive / hyperreactive / intolerant
Eyes	dark circles / puffy / redness

Summary

Skin type   normal / dry / oily / combination / sensitive

Skin condition / s to treat (from information gathered above):

_____

_____

Proposed treatment plan

Superficial cleanse	Skin analysis	Deep cleanse	Exfoliation
Skin warming	Extraction	Facial massage	Mask

Specifics of treatment plan – any adaptations required / specialised products or services to be added to the treatment plan:

_____

_____

_____

Skin analysis and skin typing

It is important for clients to realise that the skincare products they use can affect the skin's dryness, oiliness and sensitivity. The wrong choice of skincare products can trigger allergies, redness and changes in skin texture, and can aggravate breakout.

Clients often assume that once their skin type has been analysed, it will be the same forever. Physical changes, emotions, weight fluctuations, stress, hormone levels, lifestyle and the weather can all affect the skin so a client's skincare routine should not focus on skin type alone but should also consider these other factors. It is not unusual for clients to have a little bit of each skin type simultaneously, or at different times of the month.

Clients may also need to use separate products to deal with different skin types on the face, as it is important to treat different skin types, even on the same face, differently. It is imperative for skincare therapists to pay attention to the condition of the client's skin at the time of their facial treatment.

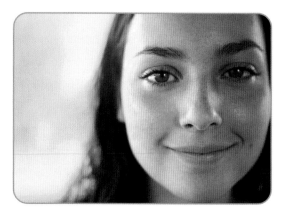

Teenagers often have combination skin

Treatment planning for specific skin types

The process of a facial treatment involves many detailed steps, as discussed in Chapter 7, which once mastered, may be adapted in terms of product choice and mode of treatment to suit the individual client's needs. Different skin types will pose different challenges to the facial therapist, and certain steps or procedures may be added, or omitted from the basic protocols, based on the skin type and condition presented.

Depending on the skincare products the skincare professional chooses, there are likely to be signature treatments and products in the range which are designed to suit specific skin types/conditions, and for which the therapist will receive additional training.

In this section we explore some general guidelines as to the considerations in adapting the facial treatment programme to suit the needs of different skin types and conditions.

Treatment planning for dry skins

A significant factor in the treatment of dry skin is to maintain the health of the skin's intercellular matrix. When skin becomes dry it is not that it lacks water, but rather that it lacks the ability to prevent water loss, or to keep the correct amount of water in its cells. Disturbance of the intercellular matrix impairs the health of the skin's cells and its layers become dry, torn and flaky.

Factors to consider in the treatment of dry skin

✂ Avoid any products with harsh, drying or irritating ingredients that are likely to disrupt the intercellular matrix.

- The use of gentle exfoliants such as enzyme peels and gentle AHAs can help to exfoliate the dead skin cells and help restore the intercellular matrix.
- Use a nourishing cream or a more penetrating serum in the facial massage.
- Use a non-setting (ideally cream or gel) mask.
- Use emollient moisturisers with lipids and natural moisturising factors (such as hyaluronic acid and ceramides).
- Advise clients with dry skin to avoid immersing their skin in water for prolonged periods of time.

Treatment planning for oily or blemished skins

The primary consideration with oily skin is to focus on deep cleansing the skin.

Factors to consider in the treatment of an oily skin

- Use water-based products and avoid any heavy products that may have a tendency to clog the pores.
- Although oily skin can usually tolerate more stimulation and harsher products, care needs to be taken to avoid overdoing the stimulation or the skin may become dry.
- A slightly more abrasive exfoliator, such as a scrub, will help to keep the follicles clean and prevent sebum and cells from building up.
- Absorbent face masks are better suited to help absorb excess oil.
- Advise clients with an oily skin to use a moisturiser only in the dry areas of their face.

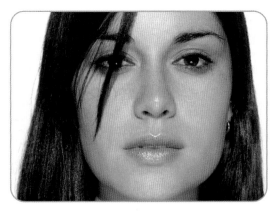

Mediterranean-type skin tends to be oily

Treatment planning for ageing/mature skins

It is important to realise that although the appearance of a client's skin may be improved with the right products and treatments, the ageing process cannot be reversed.

The barrier function decreases with age and cumulative sun damage. When the skin has a poor barrier function, water escapes from the lower levels and irritants can penetrate the skin much more easily, causing inflammation and free radical damage. Another major factor in the ageing process is the hormone loss (reduction in oestrogen levels during the menopause).

Factors to consider in aiding skin rejuvenation in ageing/mature skins

- Use products with antioxidant ingredients, and remember that antioxidants may be incorporated into the daily diet by eating foods high in vitamins C, E and A.
- The use of AHAs can help to reverse the effects of sun damage by facilitating cellular renewal and repair, thus

improving the appearance of lines and wrinkles.

- Concentrate on hydrating the skin, by using products with hydrating ingredients that help to retain moisture.
- Use a nourishing cream or a more penetrating serum in the facial massage, as with the treatment of dry skin.
- Take care to support the skin fully when carrying out the facial massage.
- Advise clients to protect the barrier function of the skin and avoid sun exposure, and to wear a sunscreen daily.

Treatment planning for skins with acne

The first consideration in the treatment of a client with acute or chronic acne is whether they need a referral to a medical practitioner and/or dermatologist. In some cases, without medical intervention to treat the bacteria trapped inside and blocking the follicle, no amount of diligent work by the skincare therapist or specialist products will really help to clear the condition.

Factors to consider in the treatment of a skin with acne

- Cleanse the skin gently with a water-based cleanser that does not contain ingredients that are likely to clog the pores or irritate the skin (avoid cleansers that are too emollient and leave a greasy film on the skin). Products for acne-prone skins often contain agents that help to control oil and remove excess sebum, along with agents that help to reduce redness and irritation.
- Avoid irritating the skin by the overzealous use of products such as cleansers and exfoliants, which will make

the skin appear redder, more irritated and more swollen.

- Encourage healthy skin turnover and removal of dead skin cells with the use of gentle exfoliants (scrubs will tend to be too irritating on inflamed areas).
- Avoid any pressure massage movements in the facial massage; light massage may be applied to areas that are not inflamed.
- Advise the client to eliminate the use of all comedogenic products.
- Avoid self trauma (i.e. scratching or picking at lesions).

Treatment planning for sensitive skins

An important consideration when treating sensitive skin is to bear in mind that the barrier of the skin is thinner and more fragile than with any other skin type, and anything that is applied to the skin will not only penetrate faster, but more of it may penetrate into the skin and cause a reaction.

As blood vessels and nerve endings are closer to the surface, sensitive skin is more likely to react to more stimulating or aggressive forms of treatment, therefore it is best to consider the following guidelines when treating sensitive skin.

Factors to consider in the treatment of a sensitive skin

- Try the simpler and gentler forms of treatments first to assess how 'reactive' the skin is.
- Use a gentle cleansing milk, and avoid any products which may strip the skin's barrier protection (for instance, detergent-type cleansers/exfoliants, products with drying alcohols).

- If exfoliating sensitive skin, it is best to use an enzyme peel and avoid any harsh abrasive forms of exfoliation.
- Use products with ingredients that are calming to the skin and are likely to decrease inflammation (gel masks are often the best type of masks for sensitive skins).
- Avoid all known sensitisers and irritants, and use a product range designed and tested specifically for sensitive skins which will protect the lipid and barrier function of the skin.
- Avoid the use of heat and steam in the treatment.
- Avoid using too much stimulation when massaging the skin.

Treatment planning for pigmented skins

Pigmented skin is one of the most difficult types of skin to treat, as there are so many variables in the causes of pigmentation, such as hormones, sun damage and ethnicity.

- Advise the client to avoid sun exposure and to wear a sunscreen every day.
- Avoid any form of treatment that is likely to increase the stimulation of melanocytes (such as overuse of exfoliants, an over-aggressive microdermabrasion treatment, or any other form of treatment that leaves the skin very irritated).
- The use of AHAs and peels may help to reduce some of the hyperpigmentation.

Facial products and treatment record

The final step in the consultation is recording the treatments and products used in the salon, and any products purchased for home use.

It is helpful to give the client a Product Prescription Card, listing the recommended products and method and frequency of use.

facials and skincare in essence

FAQs: Client consultation and skin analysis

Are there any precautions that should be taken into account when treating a pregnant client?

Most facial applications can usually be carried out safely and routinely on a pregnant client, apart from electrical treatments, which should be avoided. Due to the increased blood supply during pregnancy, some clients may find their skin has increased sensitivity, which may lead to enlarged capillaries on the face. It is best to avoid any products and applications that are considered to be more stimulating to avoid any adverse reactions. If clients develop areas of hyperpigmentation do not treat these during pregnancy as they usually fade shortly after the birth.

Why is a hormonal implant considered to be a localised contraindication?

Wherever they are situated, hormonal implants may increase the skin's ability to absorb products. This makes the area potentially more vulnerable and sensitive to reactions from products, even if a client's skin has never reacted before.

Is it possible to carry out a facial on a client who has a musculo-skeletal disorder (such as arthritis, rheumatism, spondylitis, osteoporosis or whiplash) or is it best to avoid treatment altogether?

It is usually possible to carry out some form of facial massage by adapting the treatment, but it is best for a client to seek medical advice in cases where pain and discomfort are severe. Care would need to be taken to avoid forcibly mobilising ankylosed joints, as excessive movement and pressure may cause joint pain and damage. If a joint was acutely inflamed, then any form of stimulation would need to be avoided. Gentle massage may help to ease pain, and care should be taken to position the client according to individual comfort (extra cushioning and support may be required).

Can you explain why nervous system disorders could affect the provision of facial treatment?

Nervous system disorders can be complex in nature and require medical advice in order to ascertain the potential risks. In the case of a client with a nervous disorder, it is important to know the history of the client's condition and whether they are taking medication to control any symptoms. It is important to be aware of any significant triggers in order to avoid any adverse reactions during a treatment. In the case of clients with epilepsy, some may have temporary seizures or brief spells of unconsciousness, which will present a safety risk. Some nervous system disorders may present loss of sensation and in some cases massage may trigger muscle spasms.

At what point does recent scar tissue cease to be a localised contraindication?

Scar tissue is the result of the skin's repair process for wounds and should be treated as a localised contraindication until the wound has healed. Once the scar tissue starts to form, light massage may be performed around the area in order to accelerate the repair process. Remember that the more the skin is damaged, the longer it will take to heal and each client's scar tissue should be assessed individually.

Is it true that you can shrink the size of a pore?

No, as the sizes of the pores are genetically determined. Pores may become enlarged if they are impacted with keratin, sebaceous material or bacteria. However, alpha hydroxy acids can help break up these materials and return pores to their original size.

facial product knowledge

The skincare industry is constantly developing new products to help improve the appearance of the skin. Skincare products work by chemical reactions; in order to carry out an effective facial treatment it is important to understand how products react with the skin to achieve the desired results.

The main components

The ingredients used in skincare products may be classified in two ways: functional and performance.

- Functional ingredients make up the bulk of the product and give it a specific form, such as a cream or a lotion.

- Performance ingredients aim to change the appearance and texture of the skin, and are often referred to as the 'active agents' or 'actives'.

Oil and water

Almost all skincare products are made up of oil and water and may be an oil-in-water emulsion (oils suspended in a water base) or a water-in-oil emulsion (droplets of water are suspended in an oil base).

Oil-in-water emulsions contain a small amount of oil and a greater amount of water. Examples include cleansing or moisturising lotions.

Water-in-oil emulsions contain a smaller amount of water and a greater amount of oil and are therefore heavier in consistency. Examples include cleansing or moisturising creams.

A wide array of oils are used in skincare products, which vary in their fat content, heaviness and thickness. Oils may be sourced from the earth (as in mineral oil), or from plants (common examples are jojoba, coconut and sunflower oils).

As the skin has a high water content, it comes as no surprise that water is one of the most commonly used ingredients in skincare products. Water acts as a vehicle, keeping all the other ingredients in solution, and helping to distribute the product across the skin. In terms of performance, water helps to replenish moisture in the surface epidermal layers. On a product ingredient label water is listed as *aqua*.

Product ingredient labels

A product ingredient dictionary is an essential resource for a skincare therapist. It lists the properties of natural and synthetic ingredients used to make up facial products. Some ingredients are more likely to cause skin reactions than others so it is very important to be aware of a client's allergies and the ingredients used in the treatment in order to avoid problems and adverse reactions.

Knowing the main components of the product will help the therapist understand the overall performance of the product. Ingredients are required by law to be listed in descending order of weight: the further down the list, the smaller the proportion of the ingredient is. A good rule of thumb is to divide the ingredients list into thirds: the top third usually contains 90–95 per cent of the product, the middle third usually 5–8 per cent, and the bottom third 1–3 per cent.

Cleansing agents

The active agents in cleansers are either detergents or emulsions.

Detergent

A detergent is a type of surfactant (a chemical that reduces the surface tension between the skin and the product) aiding the distribution of the product across the skin's surface. Detergents (for example, sodium lauryl sulfate) cause the cleanser to foam in use.

By reducing the surface tension detergents effectively remove dirt and oil from the skin. If detergents are too strong they may remove too much oil and damage the protective barrier.

For sensitive and dry skins manufacturers often add a fatty acid, oil or wax to reduce the contact of the surfactant with the skin to minimise the risk of irritation or dehydration. Surfactants may also be added to creams in order to improve their slip and adhesive qualities.

Emulsion

Emulsion cleansers are commonly known as cleansing milks. They are made from mostly water, with an oil or fat mixed in (oil-in-water emulsion).

The oil or fat in the emulsion is the active agent, creating a slippery surface for the removal of make-up and cell debris from the skin's surface. As cleansing milks tend to leave a slightly oily residue on the skin, emulsion cleansers should always be followed by the use of a toner.

An emulsifier is a compound added to an emulsion to help the drops to disperse, thereby keeping water and oil solutions well mixed. Glyceryl stearate, butyl stearate, polyethylene glycol and beeswax are all examples of emulsifiers used in skincare products.

Toner ingredients

The pH scale determines whether a product is acid or alkaline. Acids have pH values less than 7.0 and alkalines have pH values higher than 7.0.

The pH of the skin is between 4.5 and 6.2 and is therefore acidic. The barrier on the surface of the skin, formed by sebum and sweat, is known as the acid mantle. This forms a protective barrier against bacteria and micro-organisms. Most toners have a low pH, usually around 4.0 to 5.5, to help to restore the normal pH of the skin's acid mantle after cleansing.

Toners vary according to the skin type they are designed for. Toners for oily skins act as astringents that are said to have a tightening effect on the skin or pore appearance. Common astringent ingredients include witchhazel and citrus extracts. Toners for dry skins contain humectant ingredients to help retain and attract moisture; examples of these are butylene glycol, propylene glycol and sorbitol.

Alcohols

Alcohols are often used in toners for oily skins. Isopropyl and SD alcohols are examples of drying alcohols and, although large amounts of these would be irritating or overdrying to the skin, they may be helpful for removing excess quantities of sebum.

There are also many types of fatty alcohols used in skincare products to help improve the viscosity of lotions and creams; examples include cetyl alcohol and stearyl alcohol. Compounds listed with an –ol ending may be recognised as alcohols on an ingredient listing.

Hydrating and moisturising agents

Most moisturising products are a combination of emollients and humectants.

Emollients

Emollients are fatty substances with a lubricating action which condition the skin and provide a barrier function. Emollients lie on the surface of the skin and help prevent dehydration by trapping water to increase water retention in the epidermis. A common example of emollients used in skincare is fatty acids, such as linoleic acid, derived from plant sources including sunflower, evening primrose or borage oil. They help give a firm texture to lotions and creams. Cocoa and shea butter are other examples of natural emollients.

Fatty esters, such as glyceryl stearate, propylene glycol and cetyl palmirate, are used in skincare mainly as emollients, as they smooth the surface of the skin and serve as a protectant. One of their best qualities is that they feel less oily to the touch than some other types of fatty ingredients. Fatty esters generally have the suffix '–ate'.

Humectants

Humectants, or hydrators (also known as hydrophilic, meaning water-loving), are ingredients that are used to attract water to the skin's surface. By attracting and locking water on to the skin, humectants improve skin hydration. Humectants used in skincare include sodium hyaluronate, glycerin and panthenol (pro-vitamin B5).

Other agents found in skincare products

Solvents

Solvents are used in skincare products to act as vehicles for other ingredients. A solvent is a chemical substance used to dissolve, suspend, or extract other materials, usually without a chemical change taking place in either the solvent or the other materials. Alcohols of various types are often used as solvents for plant extracts.

Preservatives

Preservatives have an important function in skincare products in that they prevent the growth of bacteria that may be harmful. Common examples of preservatives used in products include butylparaben, ethylparaben and propylparaben. They also help protect the ingredients from chemical changes that could affect the action of the product. Products containing extracts of essential oils are considered to have their own natural preservatives as many are antiseptic in nature.

Antioxidants

Antioxidants, such as tocopherol (vitamin E) and benzoic acid, are chemicals which prevent or slow down oxidation which can cause products to develop colour and odour changes. A product which has oxidised is said to be rancid.

Colour

Many skincare manufacturers eliminate colour from their products, as some colouring agents can cause allergic reactions. Colour is only added to make the product more aesthetically pleasing, and natural or synthetic colourings may be used. Colour may be provided by the ingredients used to make up the product: blue chamomile in a cleanser gives the product a natural blue colour.

Fragrance

Fragrance, obtained from plant, animal or synthetic sources, may be added to enhance the aesthetic appeal. Essential oils or plant extracts are frequently used as their aroma is highly concentrated and they have properties which can contribute to the overall action of the product (for example, to relax or enliven the skin).

Skincare product legislation

The legislation that exists regarding the regulation of skincare products is the Cosmetic Products (Safety) Regulations 2004 (amended in 2005). Under this legislation skincare products are defined as cosmetics due to their function (which may be to clean, perfume, change the appearance, protect or maintain condition) and their field of application (via the epidermis).

The Cosmetic Regulations require all cosmetic products to be marked with:

- A full list of ingredients.
- Name and address of the manufacturer or supplier.
- Date of minimum durability (best before date).

- Warning statements and precautions.
- Batch number or lot number.
- Product function, when appropriate.

In addition to the aforementioned there should be a declared quantity of the contents, required under the Weights and Measures Act, and all lettering must be visible, indelible and easily read.

Claims in cosmetics

As a skincare therapist, or aesthetician, it is important to be careful about information you give clients about products. Avoid making claims that a product affects the physiology of the skin. Careful choice of words is needed to avoid making unqualified statements such as, 'This product reduces the appearance of fine lines'.

> Note The Cosmetics Directive bans the testing of finished products on animals in any territory of the EU from September 2004.

Useful websites to keep up to date with any changes to the legislation of cosmetics and skincare products are:

- Department of Trade and Industry (DTI) **www.dti.gov.uk**
- European Cosmetic Toiletry and Perfumery Association (Colipa) **www.colipa.com**
- Cosmetic Toiletry and Perfumery Association Ltd (CTPA) **www.ctpa.org.uk**

Facial products: types and uses

Cleansers

Cleansers remove stale make-up, dirt and excess surface secretions such as sebum, sweat and dead skin cells, along with some associated bacteria and fungi.

Skincare products and further treatment applications will not be effective if there is make-up or other residual surface matter left on the skin. If stale make-up, dirt and surface secretions build up on the surface of the skin they prevent efficient function and desquamation, block the pores, cause irritation and can eventually lead to the formation of blemishes.

Cleansing creams

These are generally used for a dry and/or mature skin and are available in a range of consistencies and textures. Normally water-in-oil emulsions, some creams are oil-in-water formulations. The oily materials dissolve the base and pigments in the make-up, lifting it and any dirt or grime from the skin's surface. Applied to the face and neck with the pads of the fingers, using gentle upward circular movements, they become more fluid at body temperature and spread easily over the skin. Thorough toning is required to avoid leaving traces of cream in the pores.

Cleansing milks

These are available in many consistencies. Most milks are emulsions and are made of differing proportions of water and oil, but contain more water than a cream. They usually have a small amount of detergent added.

79

They are suitable for removing light make-up or for cleansing a skin without make-up. Those containing a detergent element are good for oily or seborrhoeic skin and help remove surface blockages. Some contain extra emollients to avoid a drying effect.

Cleansing milks may be suitable for a mature client who wears little or no make-up and prefers the feel of a milk to a cream. They are ideal for younger skins as they do not feel greasy and are more easily removed.

They are either applied directly to the skin with clean, damp cotton pads stroked firmly but gently over the face and neck in upward and outward movements, or applied with clean fingers in small, gentle circular movements.

Cleansing lotions

Generally solutions of detergent in water, some contain antibacterial agents for oily, blemished skin. They are only recommended for use on oily or blocked skin due to their powerful degreasing action. They are not suitable for removing make-up. They tend to be preferred by young clients because they provide a clean, fresh feeling.

Soapless cleansers

Soapless cleansers can be liquid, semi-liquid or soap bars, which are compressed blocks of cleansing cream containing a soapless detergent. They lather up with water and feel the same as soap, without the undesirable side effects. Having a milder action than soap, they aim to clear surface oils and correct the pH balance, unlike soap which can cause the skin to become over-alkaline and feel taut.

Soapless cleansers can be used to wash the face after removing make-up with another cleansing product but must be rinsed off thoroughly. They are the ideal choice for those clients who like the feel of having washed their face, and they are particularly effective for oily, seborrhoeic and acned skins.

Toners

Toners remove residual grease and cleanser. They have an astringent effect, which cools, freshens and refines the skin. Toning products normally contain alcohol, which helps to restore the acid balance of the skin after washing or cleansing. As the alcohol evaporates from the surface of the skin the superficial blood vessels contract, making the skin feel cold. The strength of a toner depends on the amount of alcohol it contains. Skin tonics and astringents generally contain up to 35 per cent, whereas a skin freshener will only contain up to 10 per cent.

Skin freshener

A skin freshener has a mild, gentle action so they are suitable for use on dry or sensitive skin. The lower concentrations of alcohol in these products make them less efficient at removing grease. The basic ingredient is often a flower water, such as rose water or orange flower water. Other soothing ingredients may be incorporated, such as azulene, camomile and allantoin.

Skin tonic

A skin tonic is slightly stronger than a skin freshener but it is still quite mild in effect. Depending on its formulation it can be suitable for use on dry, delicate, dehydrated, mature or normal skins. Tonics are essentially based on alcohol but rarely contain more than 10–15 per cent. A tonic that contains more than 25 per cent alcohol should be restricted to use on greasy skin as serious dehydration could occur if used on dry skin.

Astringent

The drying and stimulating action of an astringent limits its use to combination, oily, coarse, problem skins with no evidence of sensitivity. An astringent removes surface oil and can disturb the pH balance so its use is contraindicated on delicate or dry skins due to the risk of skin irritation. Astringents are based on alcohol or compounds of boric acid or zinc plus water and other soothing additives, like glycerine, to make the product less harsh and drying. An example of an astringent is witch hazel.

> Note Astringents have a tightening effect so they should not be used on areas containing blocked pores.

Corrective/acne lotion

Excessively oily or blemished skin conditions require a corrective or acne lotion. These lotions dry and heal pustules, remove oily matter and help prevent comedone formulation. They may be diluted to help reduce their strong action if required when using on different areas of the face. They are usually chemical formulations of a spirit base with the addition of antiseptic elements to counteract infection. An excellent antiseptic ingredient for reducing follicular blockages is salicylic acid.

> Note Stronger toning lotions are required for removing excess cream (i.e. a water-in-oil emulsion) from the surface of the skin. Milder ones can be used to simply freshen the skin when there are no greasy barriers.

Exfoliators

Exfoliation is the method by which skin cells are removed from the outermost layer of the epidermis.

The effects of exfoliation are to:

- Improve skin texture and colour by removing dead skin cells.
- Remove skin blockages.
- Increase cellular regeneration.
- Increase the absorption of products into the epidermis.
- Improve the skin's ability to retain moisture.

Exfoliation may be achieved by mechanical or chemical means.

- Mechanical exfoliation removes the dead corneocytes from the top layer of the epidermis. This may be achieved through scrubs, gommages/enzyme peels or may be achieved by microdermabrasion (which is discussed in Chapter 8).
- Chemical exfoliation uses chemicals such as alpha hydroxy acids (AHAs) to loosen dead skin cells from the skin's surface.

Exfoliating ingredients

Common ingredients include polyethylene and ground nuts, such as almonds. Chemical exfoliants may contain AHAs such as glycolic acid. Certain plant extracts, such as lemon, also contain AHAs and are often added to loosen the dead skin cells. Enzyme peels containing ingredients such as papain (from the papaya fruit) help to speed up the breakdown of the protein keratin in the skin.

Exfoliants are used in a facial after the deep cleanse if the skin is congested, has a rough texture or requires the extra stimulation. All skins will benefit from at least weekly use of an exfoliating product to brighten the complexion and refine the texture of the skin. The rate of cell renewal slows with age and a more mature skin should regularly receive a gentle peeling cream to ensure a fresh appearance.

Other products and treatment applications will be accepted far more readily on a well desquamated skin.

facials and skincare in essence

> Note Although exfoliation can help cell renewal it is important to advise clients to avoid over-exfoliation. Excessive exfoliation can destroy part of the skin's natural barrier, making it subject to increased irritation and sensitivity.

Mechanical exfoliation

Scrubs

Scrubs are granular and loosen the dead skin cells by friction. They are popular with clients as they feel the scrub really is removing dead skin cells. The ingredients range from natural substances such as oatmeal, ground almonds, jojoba beads and other grains, to the more high-tech polypropylene balls.

> Note In the salon, exfoliation using scrubs may be enhanced by the use of a brush cleansing machine and the addition of steam to aid gentle but effective removal of dead cells.

Depending on the manufacturer and ingredients, scrubs may be suitable for use on all skin types, although the more abrasive are more suited to coarser/oilier skins.

Gommage/peeling creams

Gommage, meaning 'to erase', comes from the French. A creamy product applied to the skin by hand or brush, it is allowed to become slightly dry before being removed from the skin in a rolling action. Gommages may also involve the use of enzymes that help to speed up the breakdown of the protein keratin in the skin.

Depending on the manufacturer, gommages may be suitable for use on all skin types although they tend to be preferred for normal, dry or mature skins.

> Note It is important to avoid using scrubs or gommages over areas of sensitivity, redness or inflammation.

Chemical exfoliation

One of the most popular forms of chemical exfoliation carried out in salon is a fruit acid peel or AHA exfoliation treatment. It is an advanced procedure and is one that requires further training.

Fruit acid peels contain alpha hydroxy acids derived from natural sources such as citrus fruits. They gently soften and remove dead skin cells, making the skin look smoother, brighter and softer. Alpha hydroxy acids are thought to work by loosening the chemical bonds between the dead skin cells. For more information on methods of chemical exfoliation see Chapter 8.

Moisturisers

Moisturisers provide a barrier on the skin, preventing water evaporation and allowing the lower layers to rehydrate the upper layers to maintain an adequate water balance. The suppleness of the skin is therefore maintained, so delaying the ageing process and the formation of tiny lines. A barrier is also provided against the elements (sun, wind, cold and central heating).

Moisturiser also provides a base for make-up, evening out the texture of the skin and providing a smooth surface. It helps to fix the make-up on the skin, increasing its longevity. A moisturiser will prevent penetration of pigmented products into the pores, acting as a barrier between the skin and make-up so cleansing is easier. It also guards against colour change in foundations and lipsticks.

The most important ingredient of a moisturiser is water. Moisturisers are oil and water emulsions usually containing fatty materials, such as almond oil, olive oil, lanolin and sometimes humectant materials like glycerol.

Moisturising cream

Creams give the greatest protection and can be used on normal, dehydrated, dry and mature skins. They are not necessarily heavy, as the main ingredient is water, which evaporates to leave a film on the surface of the skin. It is this film which prevents the skin from losing moisture.

Creams contain about 60 per cent water and should be recommended when the surrounding atmosphere is dry, for example in central heating or very hot or cold weather. A dry atmosphere will take up water from wherever it can so a moisturiser must be replaced frequently to compensate for this.

Moisturising lotion/milk

These contain a much greater proportion of water, up to 75 per cent, and are more suitable for use on combination or greasy skins. The lighter texture of the cleansing milk ensures that it soaks into the skin quickly and they are often preferred by clients who do not want a greasy film left on the surface of their skin.

> Note It is important to remember that moisturisers are not 'treatment creams'. They do not add anything to the skin, they merely provide a barrier and their basic purpose is to conserve moisture.

Tinted moisturisers

These are very popular as an alternative to foundation for an even-textured skin. Ideal for use in the summer, they often contain UVA and UVB sunscreens to help protect the skin from the damaging effects of sunlight.

Sunscreens

The most important factor in choosing a sunscreen is whether it is one with a 'broad spectrum UVA/UVB protection', meaning that it screens out both the burning UVB rays, and the ageing UVA rays.

There are two kinds of sunblock available. The reflective type, which is also known as a 'physical block', contains minerals which bounce back light to stop the UV hitting the skin. The other type is a chemical sunscreen, which works by absorbing the UV light and preventing it entering the skin where it can cause damage. If clients have sensitive skin, the reflective sunblocks may be better, as the chemicals in high-factor sunscreens can irritate when they interact with the sun (some people may think they have a heat rash, when they are actually allergic to their sunscreen).

It is essential to buy sunscreens with an SPF (sun protection factor) suitable for your individual skin type (see guideline table on page 86), which offer a good level of protection, but which also contain any of the following as their active ingredients: avobenzone, titanium oxide or zinc oxide (when these ingredients are present, either alone or with other sunscreen agents they give equal protection from UVA and UVB radiation). An SPF is a measure of how well a

Skin type	Characteristics	Suggested SPF value
I	Always burns easily, never tans	25–30
II	Burns easily, tans slightly	25–30
III	Sometimes burns, tans gradually and moderately	15
IV	Burns minimally, always tans well	15
V	Burns rarely, tans deeply	15
VI	Almost never burns, deeply pigmented	15

sunscreen will protect the skin from sunburn, and therefore the higher the SPF, the better the protection.

Sunscreens should be applied 20 minutes to 1 hour before sun exposure.

Note It is important to advise clients to avoid applying a separate moisturiser to their sunscreen product (unless they are produced as a combination) as this will dilute the sunscreen, making it less effective. Remember it is difficult to judge the effectiveness of the sun protection levels of other products such as moisturisers, as they are not developed and tested to the same standards as specific sunscreen products.

Face masks

Masks can potentially have any performance ingredient blended into them, and are generally classified as setting or non-setting. A face mask is an 'intensive treatment' and is usually applied after massage in a facial, although this can vary according to the treatment and products applied. There are a wide variety of masks with many different purposes. If different conditions appear on the face, for example combination skin, then two or three masks may need to be applied. In this case always apply the mask that needs to remain on the skin the longest first.

Depending on the ingredients used, masks may:

ى Deep cleanse and draw out impurities.

ى Clear up blemishes.

ى Nourish and refine.

ى Hydrate.

ى Calm and soothe.

ى Tighten and tone.

Setting masks

Clay masks

- Deep cleanse – draw impurities to the surface of the skin as they dry and tighten.
- Stimulate the circulation and may aid skin toning as they (temporarily) contract pores of skin.
- Contain natural clay substances such as kaolin or sulphur.

Peel-off masks

Have a milder effect than clay-based masks because they are not absorbent.

Gel masks particularly suitable for mature or sensitive skins. Contain ingredients such as:
- *Collagen* which can be moisturising and tightening, and can help reduce the appearance of fine lines and wrinkles.
- *Aloe or seaweed extracts* which can be cooling (for calming sensitive skins).

Latex and plastic masks
- Tighten the skin temporarily.
- Some reduce skin temperature and feel very cool on the skin.
- Some stimulate the blood supply, causing the skin to go pink.
- Particularly suitable for dry and mature skins.

Paraffin wax masks retain their heat and warm the skin.
- Promote sweating, which deep cleanses and softens the skin.
- Stimulate the blood supply, causing the skin to go pink.
- Suitable for balanced and dry skins (they are unsuitable for sensitive skins).

Thermal masks

- Sometimes called Modellage masks.
- Deep cleansing, tightening and stimulating in effect.
- Contain mineral ingredients that are mixed to a paste and applied to the skin over a special cream.
- After a few minutes the paste begins to harden and a chemical reaction occurs between the ingredients, creating heat and warming the surface tissues.
- The heat from the mask encourages absorption of products applied underneath.
- The heat dissipates after 15–20 minutes, after which time the mask becomes rigid and may be eased away from the skin.

Non-setting masks

Cream masks

- Ready-prepared cream masks are quick, convenient and easy to apply.
- May have a cooling, refreshing and softening effect on the skin.
- As there are cream masks available for all skin types, they may be used to treat specific skin problems. It is often recommended that more than one mask is used to achieve the best results.
- Ingredients may be clay-based with emollient properties added: plant and aromatic extracts, essential oils, marine-based products and anti-ageing ingredients.

Non-setting masks *continued*

Warm oil masks	✂ Beneficial for dry and mature skins. ✂ Not suitable for clients with very sensitive skins who have dilated capillaries or high colouring.
Natural masks from fruit, plant and herbal sources	✂ Gentle but effective action on the skin. ✂ Based on natural active ingredients such as flower, herbal, plant and vegetable extracts. ✂ Common examples of ingredients include avocado, cucumber, papaya, oatmeal and camomile. ✂ Available as creams, gels or emulsions. ✂✂ Form a light film on the skin, which becomes firm but does not tighten. ✂ Biological masks may be used for a variety of purposes, depending on their ingredients (for example, to hydrate the skin, stimulate the circulation, correct the pH balance, or balance and regenerate the skin).

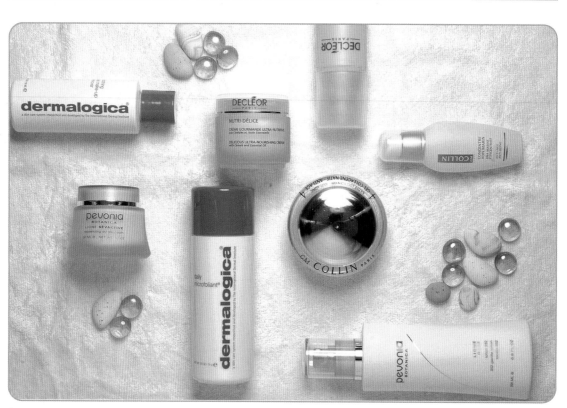

Skincare products

Specialist skincare products

The skin's appearance may be enhanced by the use of specialist products such as treatment creams, serums, ampoules, eye creams, gels and lip balms.

Treatment creams

Treatment creams tend to be heavier in consistency and texture than moisturisers and contain more emollient and active ingredients. The degree of emollient added is dependent on the skin type for which the cream is designed (treatment creams for oily skins have very little or no emollient).

Treatment creams are designed for nourishing and conditioning the skin during sleep, and may also be referred to as night creams.

Ampoules

Ampoules are produced by some manufacturers for use in facial treatments. They contain a single application of highly concentrated active ingredients in a sealed vial and are designed to address a wide range of skin types and problems. They are usually lightly massaged into the client's skin until fully absorbed, although manufacturers' instructions should be followed.

Serums

Serums are concentrates of active ingredients (typically containing vitamins, lipids and antioxidants), designed to act as 'intensive correctors' for a range of skin types and conditions. Serums are designed to be used night and day for a period of between 30 and 60 days, depending on the product and manufacturer. Designed for both salon and home use, the success of the intensive treatment relies on the client using the product correctly at home.

Eye creams

Eye creams are designed to help soften and prevent the formation of lines and wrinkles around the eyes. They contain lightweight fatty materials so that they do not stretch or drag the delicate skin when applied. Oil-in-water emulsions are absorbed easily into the skin and can be used as a base for make-up, whereas richer water-in-oil emulsions are greasier and therefore only applied at night.

Eye gels

Eye gels are designed to cool, soothe, firm and tighten the skin around the eyes. They are ideal for revitalising tired eyes and reducing the effects of fine lines by decongesting puffiness and slackness of the skin. They are basically astringents thickened with an ingredient such as methyl cellulose. Witch hazel is often used in eye gels; other ingredients that may be included are plant and herbal extracts, collagen, camomile, cornflower and azulene. Eye gels can be applied at any time of the day, though are usually used in the morning and at night.

Lip balms

Lip balms are designed to soften and moisturise to prevent the lips from becoming chapped and to help reduce the appearance of fine lines around the mouth. They also provide a good base for lipstick. Most lip balms contain emollient properties and are formed from high-melting-point hardened fat which provides a thick protective coating.

Advanced and specialist ingredients

New products with hi-tech ingredients designed to enhance the skin and improve its function, as well as address some of the major causes of ageing such as photo-damage and hormones, are being researched and developed all the time.

Note A vast array of natural and synthetic ingredients are used in skincare products, all of which will vary according to the manufacturer. It is therefore wise for therapists to research ingredients carefully for their efficacy and known benefits.

There are many examples of specialist and advanced skincare ingredients.

Antioxidants

Antioxidants are believed to be one of the most effective skin treatments (particularly for ageing or sun-damaged skin). Antioxidants are vitamins, amino acids and other natural substances, such as vitamins C, E and A, green tea and coenzyme Q10, that are thought to protect the skin by attaching themselves to free radicals and helping neutralise their damaging effects. Antioxidant ingredients help the skin cope with the effects of environmental influences.

Examples of antioxidant ingredients used in skincare products

Vitamin C (ascorbic acid)	Water soluble. Clinically proven to increase collagen production. Healing properties. Reduces fine lines and wrinkles, minimizes scars. Look for vitamin C Ester (*ascorbyl palmitate*) on ingredient labels.
Vitamin E (tocopherol)	Clinically proven to improve skin's moisture content. Has skin protection, smoothing, and healing properties. Used to help reduce the effects of free radicals formed from sun damage. Ingredient description should state high-potency E.
Vitamin A	Effective antioxidant with important rejuvenating effects on the skin. Used in anti-ageing creams known as retinoids, or vitamin A derivatives.
Coenzyme Q10	Thought to repair sun-damaged skin, energize new cell growth, possess firming properties, and smooth skin. Usually used in skin treatment creams.
Green tea	Active ingredient in many combination moisturising products. Said to be a powerful antioxidant: reduces puffiness, diminishes fine lines and wrinkles, reduces large pores, decreases inflammation and aids healing.

Examples of antioxidant ingredients used in skincare products *continued*

| **Alpha lipoic acid** | • Free radical thirst-quenching fatty acid found in every cell of the body.
• Powerful antioxidant and is claimed to have superior abilities in protecting and rejuvenating the skin. |

Peptides

Copper-peptides	• Enhance skin's protective ability, stimulate collagen formation, improve elasticity, and promote elastin production, as well as providing antioxidant and healing properties.
Pentapeptides	• Help stimulate collagen production, improve skin elasticity, repair sun-damaged skin and diminish wrinkles.
Acetyl Hexapeptide-3	• Helps smooth wrinkles by relaxing facial muscles.
Palmitoyl Oligopeptide	• Helps regenerate the skin's upper layers by stimulating collagen production and thickening the epidermis.

Examples of moisturising ingredients used in skincare products

| **Panthenol** | • Converted into vitamin B5 when applied topically to the skin: helps aid tissue repair.
• Humectant: holds water in a product, or attracts water from the environment, resulting in a penetrating moisturising effect. |

| **Ceramides** | • Naturally occurring lipids in the skin, contributing to the skin's natural moisturising factor.
• Added to skincare products to help strengthen the retention of moisture, acting primarily on the intercellular spaces of the horny layer of the epidermis where they form a protective barrier and reduce natural transepidermal water loss from the skin. |

| **Hyaluronic acid** | • A natural moisturiser that occurs in the dermis and forms part of the tissue surrounding the collagen and elastin fibres.
• Skin produces less hyaluronic acid as we age and becomes less resilient and loses elasticity.
• Added to skincare products such as moisturisers, and is used in conjunction with vitamin C to assist in maximising absorption into the skin.
• Said to improve the skin's appearance by helping to diminish fine lines and wrinkles due to its excellent water-binding capabilities.
• May also be injected by doctors into the skin. |

Examples of anti-ageing ingredients used in skincare products

| **Alpha hydroxy acids (AHAs)** | • One of the few anti-ageing treatments that have been repeatedly clinically proven as highly effective.
• Designed primarily as an exfoliant, but also stimulate skin repair, increase collagen production, increase skin thickness, improve elasticity, are effective in the treatment of acne, improve skin texture, and help improve skin tone. |

Examples of anti-ageing ingredients used in skincare products *continued*

	Note: skin needs to become accustomed gradually to AHAs due to potential irritation. High concentrations should only be utilised under the supervision of a skincare professional.
	Include glycolic acid, lactic acid, tartaric acid and citric acids.
Glycolic acid	Glycolic acid is considered to be one of the most effective AHAs.
	Derived from sugar cane.
	Used in different percentages to dissolve abnormal epidermal keratinisation and exfoliate dead skin cells.
	Employed in anti-ageing products for its ability to improve skin hydration and reduce the appearance of fine lines and wrinkles by enhancing moisture uptake and increasing the skin's ability to bind water.
Retinoic acid (tretinoin)	Derivative of vitamin A, retinoic acid was originally prescribed in high doses for the treatment of acne and keratinisation disorders.
	Proven to refine the skin, alter collagen production and reduce the appearance of wrinkles.
	Associated with a number of adverse effects including photosensitivity, skin dryness, redness and peeling.
	Anti-ageing skincare products may contain moderate and harmless proportions of retinoic acid derivatives, which will have a hydrating effect.
Liposomes	Tiny hollow spheres of lipids (fats), filled with active ingredients.
	Able to encapsulate water-soluble as well as oil-soluble substances (such as proteins and peptides).
	Due to their compatibility and affinity with cellular membranes, the ingredients held inside them can be delivered accurately into the skin and released precisely as required.
	Used in many anti-ageing treatments to facilitate the delivery of the active ingredient through the skin layers and directly to the cells.
	Improve skin hydration, reduce fine lines and wrinkles, and improve skin texture.
Nanospheres	Smaller versions of liposomes, said to penetrate deeper into the skin due to their smaller molecular size.
Polyglucans (beta-glucans)	Hydrophilic (water-loving) ingredients, able to absorb more than 100 times their weight in water.
	Natural substances derived from yeast cell walls.
	Can be absorbed into the outer layers of the epidermis due to their small molecular size and form a protective, hydrated film.
	Used in anti-ageing products to help reduce the appearance of fine lines and wrinkles by stimulating the formation of collagen.

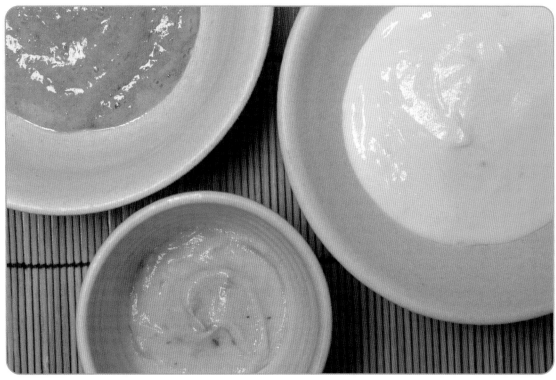

Masks made with natural ingredients

Botanical/natural extracts

There is a vast array of botanical and natural extracts found in skincare products. These may include essential oils extracted from various parts of the plant (for example, camomile, lavender, rose, sandalwood and geranium) and from the fruit (such as lemon, mango and blackcurrant). There is also a wide selection of natural carrier oils (common examples include coconut, evening primrose, grapeseed, jojoba, soya bean, avocado and borage oils) which are used to add lubricating and moisturising qualities to skincare products.

Other examples of botanical extracts used to add effectiveness to skincare products include:

Ginkgo biloba extract

Considered to be an effective anti-ageing ingredient due to its antioxidant properties, and the fact that it is said to aid fibroblast cells in the dermis in the production of collagen and elastin.

Ginseng extract

Associated with skin rejuvenation, ginseng extract's active components ginsenosides are said to be responsible for the revitalisation of epidermal cells.

Spirulina extract

Spirulina is a blue algae extract added to anti-ageing products as it is said to have a hydrating effect on the surface layers of the skin. It is also associated with tissue regeneration and with improving the appearance of prematurely aged skin and lines and wrinkles.

Liquorice extract

Considered to be an anti-irritant and may be used in facial products designed for sensitive skin. It is also said to be effective at reducing pigmentation.

Aloe vera

Humectant, providing moisture replacement, healing and soothing.

Choosing a product line

One of the most important decisions in offering a professional skincare service is which product line to choose.

There is a large selection of skincare products available and when choosing products it is helpful to consider the following:

- What type of market do you wish to attract?
- What are the initial start-up costs, trade and retail pricing?
- What are the active ingredients of the products (in other words, what results can you expect)?
- Is there an extensive range (i.e. is it suitable for all skin types/needs)?
- Is the product line recognisable and reputable within the skincare industry?
- How is the product packaged? Is it attractive enough to enhance retail sales?
- What support you can expect from the company (such as marketing and promotional support, samples, etc.)?
- What training and development opportunities are there to help you promote the product?
- What are the terms and conditions of business (minimum order, placing of orders, deliveries, returns policy, payment terms)?

FAQs: Product knowledge

I am confused as to which facial product line to buy, as there are so many to choose from. Where do I start?

Firstly, do some research and obtain information from several skincare companies. Use the internet or the beauty magazines (see 'Where to go from here'). Don't forget to ask for samples, and once you have received the information try the products on yourself and on people whose opinion you value. Once you are convinced as to the quality and performance of the product, you then need to consider price, how the product is presented, the level of service and support offered by the company and whether you will receive any training. Getting the opinion of a therapist who is already using the product is helpful. Also consider that you may need to invest in more than one line to meet all of your clients' needs.

Is it worth investing in a product line specifically for men?

It really depends on your client market. It is becoming more and more commonplace for men to visit a salon or skincare therapist for facial treatments. Factors to take into consideration are that men generally prefer simple routines and as few products to use as possible (for instance, a foaming cleanser that also gently exfoliates and a light moisturising cream would be ideal for most

men). Before deciding to invest in a line for men, consider the packaging of your main line: if it is too feminine in colour and packaging, or in aroma, it may be off-putting to some male clients.

Is it a myth that products that are free from alcohols are better for the skin?

Alcohols have gained an undeserved bad reputation in the skincare market because when some people think of an 'alcohol' they think only of a drying alcohol such as isopropyl. From a biochemical point of view the term 'alcohol' means that there is a molecular compound with an OH at the end of it. Therefore, there are several different type of alcohols; for example, cetyl alcohol is a fatty alcohol with emollient properties, used in lotions and creams.

If I choose to use a product made with natural, plant derived botanical ingredients will this be safer and more effective for my clients?

It is important not to assume that a natural product will have a superior action to a synthetic one, as naturally derived ingredients also have the potential to produce adverse reactions in some clients' skins. The key factor here is to research and test all products for their effectiveness and potential benefits before investing money in them.

casestudy: combination skin

Laura, 24, called into the salon to buy some products, and had mentioned on the phone that she had found it very hard to find the right products for her skin needs. Upon examination a typical problem associated with a young skin was identified: blemishes and breakout, but with dry, flaky patches. Laura was confused as to what to use. At home she used a foaming cleanser, which although it helped to control the oil in her skin, seemed to be causing the unwanted dry patches. She did not use a toner or moisturiser.

We suggested she tried a light cleansing milk with natural extracts such as lemon (to help brighten the skin and control sebum production) and verbena (to help decrease any inflammation). We also suggested she always toned her skin to remove all traces of cleanser, which if left on the skin may contribute to the breakout by clogging the pores. Finally we advised applying a light moisturising lotion to protect her skin and keep it hydrated.

This was an instant success. Changing from a foaming wash-off cleanser to a cleansing milk with a toner helped clear the blemishes more effectively, whilst using a light moisturising lotion in the areas it was needed treated the dry, flaky patches.

facial massage techniques

This chapter concentrates on the application of a basic deep cleansing facial, which is the essential first step in learning facial treatments. The products and massage methods may be varied in a facial sequence, depending on the nature and objective/s of the treatment. Once you have mastered the basic steps of a deep cleansing facial, it is a logical step to progress to more advanced and specialised treatment applications.

Types of facial treatments

Deep cleansing manual facials

A basic facial involving a superficial cleanse, skin analysis, deep cleanse, exfoliation, facial massage, masks and moisturising.

Mini-facials

These usually take approximately half the time of a full facial and will generally omit the detailed skin analysis, massage and the use of specialised products. They are ideal for a new client, or for clients with limited time.

Electrical facials

A more specialised service incorporating electrical equipment into a manual facial to enhance the effects on the skin. They may include high frequency, galvanic, micro-current or microdermabrasion.

Men's facials

A customised service addressing the needs of the male market, involving products specifically designed for men.

Specialised treatments

These may be signature treatments from a specific product manufacturer that involve specialised techniques and products to achieve a more intensive outcome.

The effects and benefits of facial treatments

- Deep cleanse the skin, helping to reduce minor skin imperfections.
- Aid desquamation to improve the appearance and texture of a client's skin.
- Increase the microcirculation to the skin, aiding the absorption of nutrients and removal of waste.
- Stimulate metabolism and regeneration of skin cells.
- Help correct and rebalance skin conditions (dryness, dehydration, oiliness, etc.) by helping to restore the skin's correct moisture balance.
- Soften lines and wrinkles.
- Relax tension in muscles.
- Relax the senses to reduce stress levels.
- Create an overall feeling of nurturing and well-being.

Preparation

> Note Before beginning it is important to prepare the resources needed to perform the facial, carry out a consultation and prepare the client by explaining the procedure fully.

Preparing the treatment area

Setting up and preparing the treatment area is an integral part of the facial service. In order to provide a professional image and service, the environment should be clean, comfortable, well equipped and relaxing.

It is important to pay attention to the following factors:

- The room should be warm and comfortable, with blankets provided for additional warmth and comfort.
- Additional supports should be offered for the client's comfort (under the neck, back and knees).
- Lighting should ideally be subdued to create a feeling of relaxation (although a magnifier/good lighting will be needed for the skin analysis).
- There should be no unnecessary noise. A peaceful atmosphere may be aided by relaxing music.

Equipment

Treatment chair/couch preparation

The client will be in a lying or semi-reclined position, with the therapist working from behind. The height of the treatment couch, or chair, should be checked before commencing. The height of the therapist's stool/chair should also be checked to ensure it is at the right height ergonomically. Facials are a relatively long service and if your working position is not correct it may cause you to develop postural problems, with tension in the shoulders and back.

> Note The facial treatment area should be well stocked and everything should be readily available to avoid interruptions once the treatment has begun.

Trolley preparation

The facial trolley should contain the following items:

- Headband/suitable head covering for client.
- High quality cotton wool pads (dampened).
- Soft facial tissues.
- Cotton buds.
- Four bowls: one for client's jewellery (best left in her handbag for security), one for cotton wool, one for mixing and one for waste.
- Disposable or sterile spatula.
- Sterile comedone extractor.
- Sterile microlance for milia removal.
- Disposable gloves.
- A jar of prepared sterilising fluid.
- Selection of skincare products to suit different skin types.
- Mask brush.
- Mask sponges.
- Hand mirror.

You will need the magnifying lamp for skin analysis. Prepare the steamer or hot towels, if required.

Client preparation

After greeting the client warmly and carrying out the consultation, prepare the client so that they feel as comfortable as possible when lying on the couch or facial chair. Jewellery should be removed from the ears and neck and placed safely with the client's belongings.

Clients wearing contact lenses should be advised to remove them prior to treatment to avoid any irritation or discomfort.

Outer items of clothing on the upper body should be removed, and a large towel, or towelling wrap, secured under the arms and around the front of the chest. Shoulder straps may be tucked into the towel so that the shoulders and neck may be accessed freely during the facial massage.

After these preparations, settle the client on the couch, wrapping her in a blanket, if required. Ensure that the back of the couch or chair is raised slightly to take strain off her neck and avoid dizziness when she rises after the treatment. Once settled on the couch the client's hair may be secured away from the face with a headband or turban.

> Note As some headbands may be tight, it may be better to use a loose towelling wrap to cover the hair. This will prevent a client experiencing a restricted feeling to the head, as well as preserving her hairstyle.

As facials usually take some time and the facial massage encourages removal of waste products, recommend that the client visits the toilet before starting.

Hygiene precautions

Hygiene is an important consideration in the facial treatment to avoid cross-infection. Good hygiene may be achieved by:

- Washing hands before and after treatment.
- Using clean towels and linen for each client.
- Checking that the client has no infectious conditions.
- Using a spatula to remove products from jars.
- Replacing tops on bottles and jars immediately after use to avoid contamination.
- Sterilising all implements before use.

97

Facial cleansing procedure

Cleansing is designed to remove all traces of make-up, surface secretions, dirt and other pollutants, and dead skin cells from the surface of the skin so the therapist can accurately assess the client's skin prior to devising the treatment plan. If permitted to build up, these materials could lead to the formation of comedones, pustules and other skin blemishes.

> Note Skin should be deep cleansed without overstimulating the surface capillaries or disturbing the delicate pH balance. Carefully select suitable products and work gently and quickly. The cleansing routine should not take longer than 10 minutes. A deep-cleansed skin will function more efficiently.

Removal of make-up: eyes and lips

Always remove eye and lip make-up first to avoid spreading these highly tinted and fine textured cosmetics to the rest of the face.

- Firstly ask the client to close her eyes.
- Work on one eye at a time.
- Apply a small amount of cleanser/eye-make-up remover over the upper part of the eyelid with small circular movements using the pad of the ring finger (avoid putting pressure on the eyeball).
- Use the non-working hand at the top of the eyebrow and forehead in order to support and 'open up' the eye tissue.
- Gently remove make-up from the upper lid by sweeping outwards using a circular dampened cotton wool pad.

- Ask the client to look up while sweeping underneath and inward toward the nose to remove make-up from below the eye.
- Place a damp folded cotton wool disc below the lashes and, using a cotton bud dipped in eye make-up remover, roll down the lashes to remove any mascara.
- Repeat the above procedure to the other eye.
- Once both eye areas have been cleansed, take a small amount of cleanser on the ring finger and apply small circular movements from one side of the lips to the other. Use a damp cotton pad to gently wipe across to remove any residual make-up.

After cleansing the eyes and lips, begin the superficial cleanse to the face.

Cleansing the face and neck

A minimum of two cleanses should always be given.

- Superficial cleansing just removes surface make-up, stale secretions and dirt. This is carried out whether a client is wearing make-up or not.
- Deep cleansing removes ingrained impurities and gently stimulates the healthy functioning of the skin. As this is a deeper routine, the blood circulation to the facial skin is increased, having a warming effect and relaxing the hair follicles and pores, aiding absorption of the cleanser so it can more effectively dissolve make-up, surface secretions and dirt.

Cleansing routines

Apply a suitable product (usually a lightweight cleansing milk) to your hands and warm before applying to the skin.

superficial cleansing

1 Apply the cleanser to the face in the following steps:

a) Clasp your fingers together at the base of the neck and unlink them as you move up the neck.

b) Clasp your fingers together at the chin and draw them outwards to the angle of the jaw.

c) Stroke palms up the face across the cheeks to the forehead (fingertips pointing downwards).

Slide hands the down the sides of the face and repeat movements a, b and c three times.

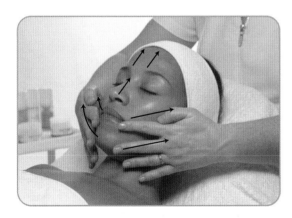

2 Using a series of light circular movements with the fingertips, work from the neck, across the chin and the cheeks, up the nose and finish at the forehead.

3 Remove the cleanser with damp cotton wool, stroking upwards and outwards in a rolling motion.

Between cleanses a mild toning lotion can be used on damp cotton wool pads to remove any greasy film from the skin.

Repeat as necessary. Depending on the amount of make-up worn by the client, more than one superficial cleanse may be needed. Repeat the superficial cleanses until the skin is free from make-up and only then move on to the deep cleanse.

Once the type and condition of the skin has been assessed, apply a suitable deep cleansing product to the skin, warming it in your hands first. The deep cleansing sequence is carried out only once.

deep cleansing

1 Repeat application, as in superficial cleansing routine (Step 1 a–c).

2 Stroke up either side of the neck (avoid pressure to the trachea and thyroid gland) using gentle pressure with the fingertips of both hands. When you reach under the chin, draw fingers outwards to the angle of the jaw and lightly stroke back down to the neck to the starting position. **Repeat x 6**

3 Apply small circular movements with the pads of the fingers over the skin of the neck (concentrating under the chin). **Repeat x 3**

4 Slide your hands up to the chin and use alternate index fingers to work up and into the crease of the chin. **Repeat x 6**

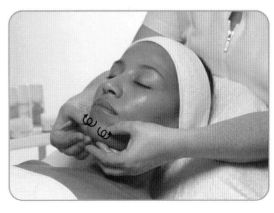

facials and skincare in essence

5 Apply small circular movements with the pad of the thumb to the crease of the chin. **Repeat x 3**

6 Apply small circular movements with the pads of the fingers over the cheeks from the corners of the mouth to the sides of the nose and up to the temples. Work back down to the corner of the mouth. **Repeat x 3**

7 Using small circular movements with the pads of the index and middle fingers, work up the sides of the nose and into the creases (taking care to avoid applying any pressure to the nostrils). **Repeat x 3**

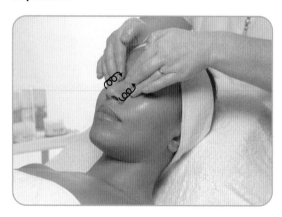

8 Using the pads of the index (or ring) fingers of both hands slide your hands up the sides of the nose. Stroke out above the eyebrows and then inwards underneath the eyes, producing a big circular movement. **Repeat x 6**

9 Using the pads of the fingers of both hands apply small circular movements across the forehead working from temple to temple (one hand following the other). **Repeat x 6**

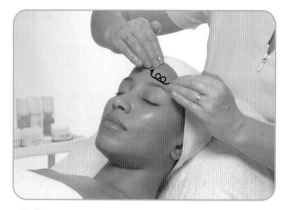

10 Using the index and middle fingers of each hand perform criss-cross/interlocking zigzag movements over the forehead. Work from one side of the temple to the other. **Repeat x 6**

11 a) Slide the index fingers of each hand under the eyes and upwards to apply gentle pressure at the start of each eyebrow.

b) Stroke the fingers across the brow line to apply gentle pressure to the middle of the brow.
c) Continue stroking the fingers across to apply pressure at the end of the eyebrow.
d) Stroke over the outer corner of the eyes and then inwards underneath the eyes towards the nose. **Repeat x 6**

12 Apply slight pressure at the temples with both palms (this indicates to the client that the cleansing sequence is complete).

13 Remove cleanser from the skin with damp cotton wool using upwards and outwards movements until the skin is completely clean.

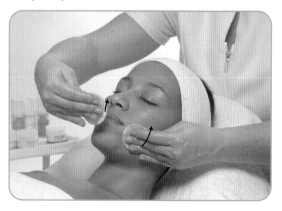

14 Tone to remove all residual cleanser.

15 Blot the skin with a tissue, if necessary (only really needed if the skin feels wet and there is excess product to remove).

Note Always take care when using a tissue to cover and blot the skin as clients who suffer with panic attacks or claustrophobia may find this procedure uncomfortable.

Exfoliation

Mechanical exfoliation is usually carried out in a deep cleansing facial. The method of application is largely dependent on the manufacturer's instructions and the client's skin type. The most popular exfoliant comes in the form of a scrub: a granular-based product used with friction.

Exfoliants are usually gently massaged into the skin, taking care to avoid the eyes and any sensitive areas. Once the product has been worked into the skin, it is then rinsed with moistened sponges or cotton pads.

Skin warming devices

Warming the skin after deep cleansing, by using steaming or hot towels, softens the pores, making it easier to remove skin blockages without damaging the surrounding skin.

Steaming

Steaming is a gentle cleansing or skin preparation treatment suitable for most skin types. It is an optional part of a facial which may be performed after deep cleansing. Some steamer models produce ozone which has an antibacterial effect and promotes healing.

Contraindications to steaming

- Extremely vascular skins.
- Clients who suffer from claustrophobia.
- Hypersensitive skins.
- Unstable skins.
- Severe bronchial conditions or asthma.
- Severe circulatory disorders.

Safety precautions

- Always refer to manufacturer's instructions.
- Use distilled water to prevent calcium and mineral deposits building up in the machine.
- Ensure the steamer has a stable base.
- Avoid placing the steamer where it is likely to get knocked.
- Keep the steam outlet directed away from the client and any other equipment/ materials while the water is heating.
- Check that an even vapour is produced before applying it to the client's face.
- Ensure the client's hair and any areas of sensitivity are protected before use.
- Keep checking the client's skin reaction during treatment.
- Turn the steam outlet away from the client before turning the machine off and move it to a safe place immediately after treatment.

101

Benefits and effects of steaming

Skin type	Benefits of steaming	Timing
Dry skin	deep cleanses, desquamates, hydrates, improves colour	5 mins
Normal/balanced skins	maintains skin function and texture, cleanses, hydrates	5–10 mins
Mature skin	increases cellular regeneration, desquamates, hydrates, improves skin colour	5 mins
Oily/combination skin	unblocks congestion, deep cleanses, improves skin colour	10 mins

Skin type	Recommended distance of steam outlet to face
Dry, mature skin	40 cms (15 inches)
Normal/balanced skin	30 cms (12 inches)
Oily skin	20 cms (10 inches)

Application

The general rule is the oilier the skin, the closer the steamer may be placed and the more sensitive the skin, the further away the steamer should be.

Any areas of sensitivity or high colour should be protected with cotton wool pads to prevent overstimulation.

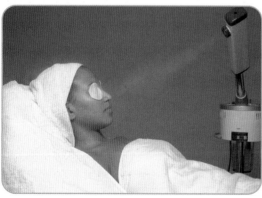

Steaming

Hot towels

Hot towels are a quick and convenient way of warming the skin. They may either be prepared with hot water from the tap, or by heating in a hot towel cabi or microwave.

Hot towels may be folded onto the client's face, pressing gently over the skin and moulding the towel to the facial contours (leaving a gap for the client's nose) and leaving it in place until heat has dissipated. The procedure may be repeated again.

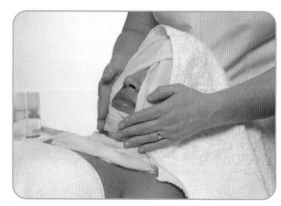

Hot towel

Extraction

Extraction, or removal of skin blockages, should always be carried out after the skin has been softened by deep cleansing or warming of the skin. Skin blockages that have been present for some time may need more steaming and skin softening before they can be released. It is important not to risk damaging the skin by attempting to force out stubborn comedones.

Extraction methods

Open comedones

It is possible to extract open comedones with the use of cotton buds, fingers around a clean tissue/cotton wool, or with a comedone extractor.

If using cotton buds it is best to use the plastic ones with a flexible stick and place a bud each side of the open comedone. Press down gently and move the cotton buds closer together with the tips touching the skin. Keep applying gentle pressure until the blockage is released. If the blockage is not released easily, reposition the cotton buds at another angle around the comedone and repeat.

If using the fingers wrapped with cotton pads/tissue use the same downward and inward pressure technique to extract the comedone. It is important to work the fingers all around the comedone and avoid using the nails to pinch and mark the skin. The advantage of using cotton buds over the fingers is that it is easier for the therapist (as they are smaller than fingers) and more comfortable for the client.

Comedone extractors are best suited to the non-fleshy parts of the face such as the forehead or cheekbones. They are only suitable for use if the blockage is smaller than the hole in the extractor. Place the extractor with the hole directly over the comedone, then apply pressure straight down on the extractor, using the leverage of the handle to extract the contents.

To avoid discomfort it is important not to apply too much pressure because the metal comedone extractor is not as flexible as fingers or cotton buds.

Closed comedones

Closed comedones may be present anywhere on the face, but are often located on the jawline, cheeks and chin.

Closed comedones are more difficult to extract. They appear as bumps under the surface of the skin and may have a very small follicle opening. If there is no follicle opening evident, then an opening must be made with a sterile microlance.

Once you have located the follicle opening to a closed comedone, place cotton swabs or buds on either side of the lesion. Gently press down on the swabs or cotton buds whilst gently turning them inwards, taking care to pull the skin taut with the outside fingers.

If the extraction method is effective a solid stream of sebaceous matter will emerge from the closed comedone.

Milia

To extract, gently spread the skin taut around the milium with your fingertips. Using a sterile microlance gently lift off the top of the cell layers of the milium, and the microlance should then slide easily into the top.

Once you have created an opening in the top of the milium, you can then apply gentle pressure on both sides of the lesion in order to release the sebaceous matter.

General guidelines

- Ensure products have been removed from the skin before commencing extraction (the face should be moist but not wet).

- Ensure the pads of the fingers/comedone extractor/cotton buds used for removing skin blockages are clean and/or sterile (therapist may wear disposable gloves).

- Avoid extracting for long periods of time (any more than 10 minutes during a treatment can be too stimulating and uncomfortable for a client).

- Keep the skin taut during extraction to reduce discomfort.

- After extraction it is advisable to wipe over the skin with a soothing antibacterial product to prevent infection.

Facial massage

The massage is usually the most favoured part of the facial service for both the therapist and the client, as it is extremely enjoyable to give and receive.

Facial massage is usually carried out using cream or oil, the choice being dependent on the client's skin type and preference. The chosen product must provide sufficient lubrication for the massage to be effectively performed and should preferably be nourishing to the skin.

Oil

As well as allowing ease of movement and deeper massage, oil nourishes and softens the skin. The oil must be light, non-sticky and easily absorbed. Pure, natural vegetable oils, such as almond, grapeseed, and peach kernel are light and easily absorbed and are beneficial to the skin.

> Note Take care to avoid all oils that are nut-based in the event of a client who suffers with a nut allergy.

Cream

There are creams available for facial massage which contain specific ingredients and are of different textures to suit all skin types. One of the most important qualities of a cream is that it is not absorbed into the skin too quickly.

Massage movements

Facial massage involves a range of massage movements which may be adapted to the client's skin type and condition, objectives of the treatment and the client's preference.

Classical massage movements used in a facial include effleurage, petrissage, tapotement and vibration.

Effleurage

Effleurage movements consist of soft, continuous stroking movements applied with the fingers and palms in a slow and rhythmical manner. They are light, even, stroking movements, which prepare the tissues for deeper massage and link up other movements in the facial sequence.

Effleurage may be applied lightly or more deeply, depending on the part being massaged and the effects required.

The effects of effleurage

- Aids desquamation to improve skin texture.

- Stimulates an increased blood flow through the superficial circulation, causing a slight increase in skin temperature.

- Soothes the nerves.

- Relaxes the client.

Petrissage

Petrissage describes a range of kneading movements that stimulate the underlying tissues. They are compression (pressure) movements used with either the whole of the palmar surface or just the pads of the thumbs and fingers.

Kneading, knuckling, rolling and pinching are examples of petrissage movements which may be included in a facial sequence. Small, deep petrissage movements are more stimulating than larger, more superficial ones.

The effects of petrissage

- Increases the circulation of blood and lymph to improve cellular nutrition and aid the removal of waste products from the tissues.
- The skin appears smooth, clear and refreshed as a result of desquamation.
- Muscle fibres become relaxed and their tone is improved.
- Eases tension nodules.

Tapotement

Tapotement is a term used to describe percussion movements, for example tapping and slapping, which are performed lightly and briskly without compressing the skin.

The effects of tapotement

- Stimulation of the superficial nerve endings causing temporary toning and tightening of the skin.
- Creates an erythema, helping to improve skin colour.
- Improved blood flow resulting from alternate constriction and relaxation of blood vessels.
- Removal of static lymph from tissues, e.g. from beneath the chin in a client with sluggish circulation.

Vibrations

Vibrations are rapid shaking movements where the muscles of the lower arms and hands are rapidly contracted and relaxed so that a mild shaking or trembling movement is produced by the fingers or thumbs. The balls of the fingertips or thumbs are pressed firmly on the point of application and the vibrations run through a nerve centre or along a nerve path, with very little surface stimulation.

The effects of vibrations

- Relaxation and relief of tension.
- Gentle stimulation of the deeper skin layers.
- Relief from muscular fatigue and pain.

Hand mobility

Facial massage techniques require extreme sensitivity and an expert touch. In order to apply facial massage effectively, a skincare therapist's hands should be flexible, supple and above all relaxed.

In order to facilitate relaxation, the hands need to maintain a regular rhythm and regulate the correct amount of pressure. Hand movements should be practised regularly so that they are smooth and glide easily from one area of the face to another, without breaking contact and thereby disturbing the client's relaxation.

Facial massage routine

Facial massage is carried out for approximately 10–15 minutes of a basic deep cleansing facial. A facial massage is usually included after all the cleansing has been carried out, and will vary according to the client and the specialised treatment provided. Techniques vary according to training and procedures established by a product manufacturer.

In general when carrying out a facial massage, bear in mind that an even rate and rhythm of movements promotes relaxation. Avoid breaking contact from the client's face once you have started, and when it becomes necessary to remove your hands feather them off gently to avoid interrupting the client's relaxation.

Illustrated below is a suggested facial massage routine, which incorporates a range of techniques which may be adapted to suit the client's needs.

Apply the chosen massage medium (cream or oil) in sweeping strokes across the décolleté and up on to the face. Each movement may be repeated up to six times

the nose and up on to the forehead). Slide the hands down the sides of the face to repeat six times; start superficially and progressively become deeper.

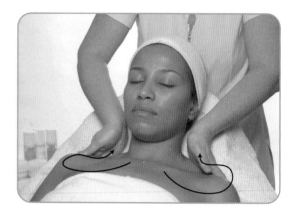

2 Place the hands either side of the sternum across the upper part of the pectoral muscles. Deep effleurage over pectorals, around the deltoids and firmly across trapezius and up the back of the neck up to the base of the skull (returning lightly down the front of the neck to the sternum).

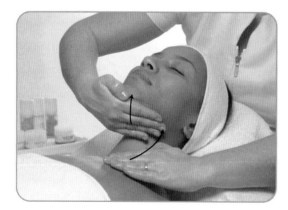

1 Use the palmar surface of each hand to effleurage in alternate sweeping strokes up the face (up each side of the neck, up from the jaw to the chin, across each side of the cheek, above lip, using the index fingers up the bridge of

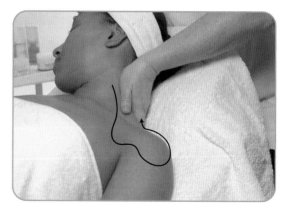

3 Turn client's head to one side (whilst still supporting the head with one hand) and use a sweeping stroke across the pectorals, around the cap of the deltoid up to the base of the skull. Then perform deep vibrations with the fingertips to the muscles in the back of the neck. Repeat on the other side of the neck

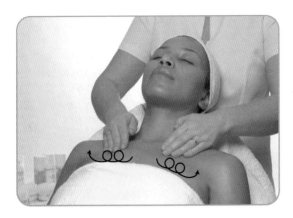

4 Use the pads of the fingers to knead in a circular motion across the pectoral muscles either side of the sternum.

5 Place each hand behind the cap of the client's shoulders and knead the deltoid muscles in a circular motion.

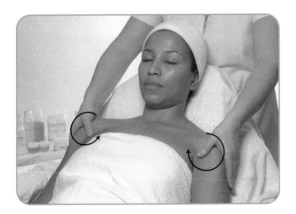

6 Use the pads of the fingers of both hands to knead the upper fibres of the trapezius.

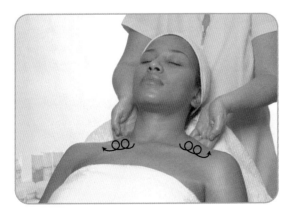

7 Use the thumbs of both hands to knead the upper fibres of the trapezius.

8 Shape both hands into loose fists and with the middle phalanges of both hands knuckle in a circular motion across the pectorals and around the deltoid to the upper fibres of the trapezius.

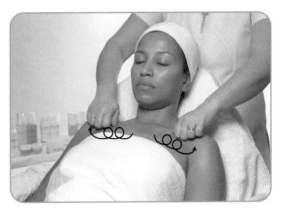

9 With a linking effleurage stroke up one side of the neck to perform cheek lifts with alternate hands on one side, then slide hands over the chin to repeat on the other side.

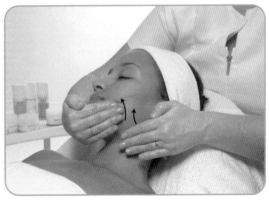

10 Thumb kneading to crook of chin, using the pads of both thumbs in a circular motion.

11 Finger kneading around the jawline in a circular motion, using both hands (one on each side of the face).

12 Finger kneading across cheeks, working from below the zygomatic up to the temple, using the pads of the fingers of both hands.

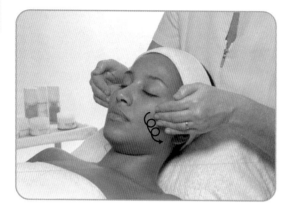

13 Knuckling across the cheek and jaw area, using the middle phalanges of both hands in a circular motion.

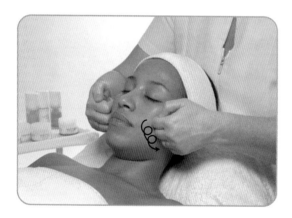

14 Slide the hands up to either side of the nose to finger knead with the pads of the index/middle fingers to either sides of the nose.

15 Slide the index fingers of both hands up either side of the nose, circle above and under the eyes, applying slight pressure at the corrugator muscle.

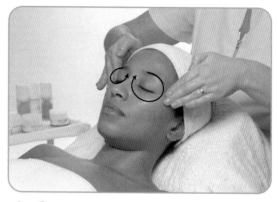

16 Using the pads of the fingers of both hands apply pressure points below the eyebrows.

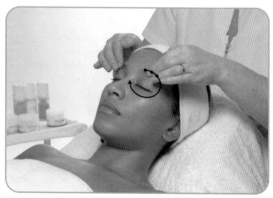

17 Place the pads of the fingers on either side of the temples and circle slowly and deeply.

18 Using the index fingers of both hands on one side of the face at a time, stroke the 'crows feet' in an upward and lifting motion with alternate fingers, then repeat on the other side.

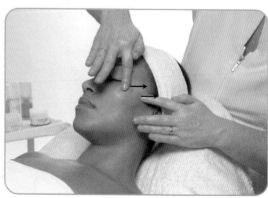

19 Circular kneading across the forehead using the pads of the fingers of both hands, working from one side of the temple to the other.

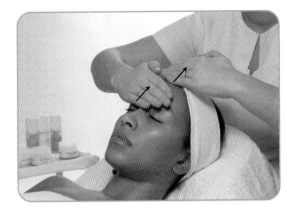

20 Place the palms of both hands just above the eyebrows and use alternate strokes firmly up the forehead.

21 Place the heels of both hands on either side of the temples and circle slowly and deeply.

22 Using a linking effleurage stroke return to the sternum to repeat movement at Step 2, gradually becoming more superficial, indicating that the massage is coming to an end.

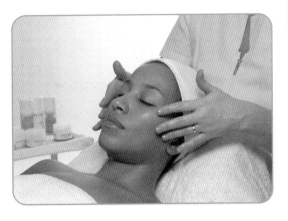

23 Apply light tapping across the face with the fingertips to gently awaken your client.

24 End with pressure on forehead with palms.

Adaptations

The skilled facial therapist must learn to adapt a facial massage to suit each individual client and their needs.

Skin type	Massage adaptation
Sluggish, lacking in tone	More stimulating massage, incorporating tapotement and vibration movements.
Dry skin	Penetrating massage with a hydrating or nourishing cream.
Delicate or sensitive	Gentler approach, using softer and gentler effleurage movements, and less pressure with petrissage movements. If dilated capillaries are present no tapotement movements would be performed.
Mature or ageing	Care taken to support the skin to avoid overstretching the tissue, and use of upward movements to help to increase tone and elasticity.
Puffy	Movements concentrating on lymphatic drainage, avoiding strong pressure which may cause discomfort.

continued

Skin type	Massage adaptation
Acned or blemished	Massage step may either be omitted to avoid overstimulation and any discomfort that may arise from the manipulation of inflamed tissues surrounding the lesions, or may be applied with less pressure and less friction over non-inflamed areas only.

Mask application

As with all other skincare products, masks are chosen according to the client's skin type and condition.

> Note In a deep cleansing facial it is common to apply a dual mask: one to treat the oilier T-zone area and one hydrating the neck and cheek areas.

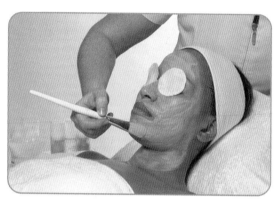

Facial mask

General guidelines

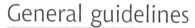

- Always follow the manufacturer's instructions regarding preparation, application and removal.
- Apply the chosen mask/s neatly and methodically, with a mask brush or clean fingers, taking care to ensure even coverage.
- If it is dual application ensure that the setting mask is applied first.
- Apply soothing eye pads once the mask application is complete.

- Time the application to ensure optimum results.

Remove masks with damp warm sponges or cotton pads using an upward motion. Repeat until all traces of the mask have been removed and finally apply a light application of toner before proceeding to the last stages of the facial.

Moisturise

The concluding step is to moisturise and protect the skin and to prevent water loss. A light application of a chosen moisturiser is applied to the face in light sweeping strokes.

At this stage a light application of eye gel or cream may also be applied, with a small tab of lip balm to nourish and protect the lips.

Contra-actions

Occasionally a client may experience an adverse reaction to a product used in a facial treatment, for instance, the skin may feel itchy and uncomfortable. If this occurs during a facial, remove all traces of the product immediately and apply a soothing lotion to cool and soothe the skin.

Always note down details of a contra-action and product reactions on a client's record card, in order to avoid any problems on a subsequent treatment.

Aftercare/homecare advice

In order that the client obtains the maximum benefit from the facial it is important that aftercare/homecare advice is given. Ideally this is best given in a written form, along with a written recommendation for the purchase of products and future treatments.

After a facial treatment the skin should be sufficiently cleansed and stimulated and is best left alone to ensure that the maximum benefit from the treatment is obtained and any contra-actions are avoided.

Dos and don'ts

- Avoid wearing make-up for up to 8 hours, except light mascara and lipstick.
- Avoid any form of direct heat or stimulation such as sauna, hot bath, hot hairdryer or ultraviolet exposure for up to 12 hours.
- Avoid swimming for up to 12 hours.
- Wear a suitable sunscreen to protect the skin.

Product and lifestyle advice

It is also important to give advice on:

- Appropriate products and how to integrate these into a homecare regime.
- Factors contributing to the ongoing health of the skin such as diet, sufficient water/fluid intake, exercise, smoking, alcohol, sun exposure, lifestyle factors and getting sufficient sleep.
- The nature and recommended frequency of future treatments.

The post-treatment consultation

Before clients leave the salon, it is the therapist's professional responsibility to educate them about maintenance of their skin, including recommending suitable products for home use.

Providing a post-treatment consultation is an essential part of a facial service as it is an

opportunity to review the client's needs based on the skin's response to the treatment and recommend an ongoing treatment plan. It is important to realise that the consultation process occurs before commencing the facial, during the facial when the skin's responses are observed, through to the post-treatment consultation when you can discuss with the client your findings and recommendations.

During the post-treatment consultation it is important to:

- Review with the client any concerns they had at the initial consultation stage; this will provide a basis for discussing your own findings.

- Provide a written recommendation of products, with specific directions for use (how, when and how much to use).

- Make suggestions about future courses of treatment and the results that can be expected.

Remember that clients' home skincare guides should be updated regularly (at least twice a year) to allow for:

- Seasonal changes.

- Changes in age and health.

- Lifestyle changes.

- New treatment/product developments.

Frequency of treatment

It is usual for clients to receive facials on a monthly basis, with use of retail products between salon visits. If a client has problem skin, initially it may be necessary for them to attend the salon more frequently (weekly or fortnightly) until the skin condition is more controlled.

Facials for men

Although a man's skincare is just as important as a woman's, it requires a slightly different approach. Although there is not specifically a 'male' skin type, it is important to consider the differences in make-up between male and female skins.

Firstly, there are hormonal differences between men and women. Testosterone, the male hormone, gives men a thicker epidermis (approximately 2 mm compared to 1.5 mm in women). Male skin does have a tendency to be tougher, more elastic and less sensitive than female skin, although daily shaving can increase the risk of skin rashes, infections and ingrowing hairs.

Male skin is also more acidic and has a more efficient supply of blood and sebum. This means it tends to age better than female skin, remaining softer, firmer and more supple.

The first consideration when providing men's facials would be to make the environment 'male friendly', avoiding the use of anything which either looks or smells too feminine.

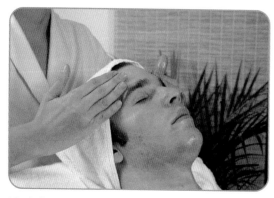

Man's facial

Adaptations

ꙮ Sponges are more suitable for use on a man's face, as cotton wool will cling to facial hair.

ꙮ Advise male clients ideally not to shave within a few hours before receiving their facial, as this will make the skin more sensitive and may contraindicate the use of certain exfoliating products.

ꙮ Apply a deeper and firmer touch for the massage elements of the facial (most male clients prefer this).

ꙮ Massage movements in the beard and moustache should be done in the direction of the hair pattern to avoid discomfort.

ꙮ Ideally use products designed for male skins; avoid using products which feel greasy on the skin, as most male clients dislike the feel of anything heavy or greasy on their skin.

ꙮ Male clients often have a preference for steaming and the use of hot towels in a facial treatment.

ꙮ Take care with any abrasive products over areas that have been shaved, as the skin will generally need calming and soothing.

Electrical treatments

Once you have learnt how to analyse skin accurately and how to apply a manual deep cleansing facial, it is a natural progression to receive training in facial electrical equipment. The following information is a brief introduction and overview of some of the more popular electrical equipment used. It is essential that therapists receive training in operating the equipment, including the safety precautions and contraindications relevant to each machine.

High frequency

High frequency uses an alternating current which passes through the skin to produce a heating, stimulating effect. A high frequency current is one which moves backwards and forwards at a very high speed, creating vibrations over the skin's surface of between 10,000 and 250,000 vibrations per second.

There are two methods of application: direct high frequency and the indirect method (known as Viennese Massage).

Direct high frequency

This uses a glass electrode which is slowly moved over the skin and the warmth generated is healing, particularly for oily, seborrhoeic skins. As this has a bactericidal effect on the skin, it is best carried out after all other applications.

Indirect high frequency

This uses a saturator which is held in the client's hand. The current is discharged through the therapist's fingers during the massage. This has a warming and relaxing effect on the client and is particularly effective for dry, dehydrated skins.

facials and skincare in essence

	Indications for use	Benefits and effects
Direct high frequency	⚲ Seborrhoeic skins. ⚲ Greasy, combinations skins. ⚲ Blemished skins. ⚲ To increase sebaceous secretions on dry, mature skin.	⚲ Warms and softens the tissues. ⚲ Produces an erythema. ⚲ Increases metabolism. ⚲ Improves skin texture. ⚲ Produces a germicidal effect. ⚲ Limits sebaceous secretions on skin's surface. ⚲ Dries and heals pustular infections.
Indirect high frequency	⚲ Dry, dehydrated skin. ⚲ Sluggish circulation. ⚲ Tired skins with fine lines. ⚲ Relaxation.	⚲ Warms and softens the tissues. ⚲ Increases metabolism. ⚲ Improves skin moisture balance. ⚲ Increases blood and lymphatic circulation.

Galvanic

Galvanic treatments use a constant direct current; one electrode is negatively charged (the cathode) while the other is positively charged (the anode).

Desincrustation

A deep cleansing treatment (chemical cleanse) to soften skin and removed hardened sebum and cell debris. It is usually carried out after deep cleansing to reinforce the general cleansing process.

Iontophoresis

The introduction of water soluble substances deep into the skin for maximum benefit. As this is a nourishing treatment, it should complete the facial routine.

	Indications for use	Benefits and effects
Desincrustation (negative pole – cathode)	⚲ General cleansing of combination and oily skin. ⚲ Deep cleansing of seborrhoeic skin. ⚲ Stimulation of sluggish skin with build up of comedones.	⚲ Produces an alkaline reaction – relaxes pores. ⚲ Stimulates nerves. ⚲ Increases blood supply. ⚲ Softens tissue. ⚲ Increases cell metabolism.
Iontophoresis (positive pole – anode)	⚲ Dry and mature skins in need of hydration and moisturising. ⚲ Mature skins in need of regeneration. ⚲ Sluggish skins in need of stimulation. ⚲ Sensitive skins may be improved with use of correct gels/ampoules.	⚲ Produces acid reaction. ⚲ Astringent effect – closes the pores. ⚲ Tightens and firms skin. ⚲ Soothes nerves. ⚲ Hardens tissue. ⚲ Refines skin texture. ⚲ Restores acid mantle.

General benefits and effects of facial galvanic

- ⚡ Vasodilation and erythema increases circulation to the face, bringing fresh oxygen and nutrients to improve the condition of the skin.
- ⚡ Increases cell metabolism to improve the condition of the skin.
- ⚡ Increased mitotic activity of the skin's cells aids desquamation.
- ⚡ Increased blood flow results in an improvement in the colour and texture of the skin.

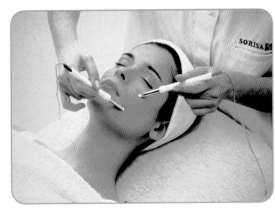
Microcurrent machine

Microcurrent

Microcurrent is used to maintain a youthful appearance and combat the effects of ageing on the skin. It offers facial (and body) contour lifting by reprogramming the muscle fibres. It can shorten or relax the fibres, thereby lifting sagging muscles of the jaw, neck and face, as well as reducing and smoothing the fine lines and wrinkles on the face and neck.

It may be offered to a wide client group, including those who wish to use the treatment as a preventative measure against premature ageing as well as to re-educate and strengthen muscles.

	Indications for use	Benefits and effects
Microcurrent	⚡ Clients wanting to maintain a youthful appearance/skin rejuvenation. ⚡ Clients with lines, wrinkles and creases. ⚡ To improve condition of ageing skin. ⚡ To improve the colour and texture of the skin to promote a healthy glow. ⚡ To reduce puffiness. ⚡ Dark circles and puffiness around the eyes. ⚡ To soften old scar tissue.	⚡ Increases cell metabolism to improve condition of skin. ⚡ Stimulates cell mitosis to enhance cell renewal. ⚡ Increases circulation to the skin, bringing more oxygen and nutrients to the cells and speeding up removal of waste. ⚡ Improves lymphatic drainage, thereby reducing puffiness. ⚡ Stimulates muscle fibres to improve muscle condition and function. ⚡ Stimulates fibroblasts to improve muscle condition and function. ⚡ Shortening of the muscles and improvement in tone.

Holistic facial massage techniques

Holistic facial massage techniques are based on the concept of achieving wellness and balance, and each method adds its own dynamic to the facial experience.

Ayurvedic facial massage

Ayurveda is recorded as the world's oldest Indian healing system. The word 'Ayurveda' comes from Sanskrit:

- Ayur = life
- Veda = knowledge

The whole aim of Ayurveda is in prevention and promoting health, beauty and long life through physical, emotional and spiritual well-being. The Ayurveda teaches that health is maintained by the balance of three subtle energies, or doshas, known as Vata, Pitta and Kapha.

An Ayurvedic facial uses the ancient principles with specific facial products to suit the client's personal dosha. In Ayurveda, a person is seen as a unique individual made up of five primary elements: ether (space), air, fire, water and earth. When any of these elements are imbalanced they will affect how an individual feels. The foods we eat and the weather are just two of the influences on these elements.

The massage in an Ayurvedic facial is a specialised marma point massage to the head, face and upper body in order to help balance a client's personal dosha, bringing them a renaissance of well-being and total rejuvenation. Marma points are the subtle pressure points, similar to acupressure points, that stimulate the life force or pranic flow. The marmas are anatomical places on the body, mostly composed of flesh and bones.

There are a total of 107 marmas in the body, 37 of which are located in the head and neck.

Marma points are naturally sensitive points that are measured by finger widths, known as anguli. The finger width is the finger of the person being treated and not the therapist's own finger. The locations of marmas are given in this way because each person has a different size and proportion. The location of marmas may vary from one to eight finger widths, and often relate to regions of the body and not a point.

Marma points may be treated with pressure, circular massage, heat and oils. The marma is first located by finding a hard, tender or sensitive point. When enough pressure has been applied, small circular movements may be used to break up the tension from the point – use circular anticlockwise movements spiralling out to the periphery; from the periphery change to clockwise movements back towards the centre.

In general clockwise movements stimulate or energise a marma point and a counterclockwise movement dispels and liberates blocked energy.

Benefits
- Releases muscles and connective tissue over the scalp and face.
- Relaxes and restores the areas around the forehead, eyes, nose and mouth.
- Eases neck and shoulder tension.
- Relaxes and uplifts the facial muscles.
- Imparts a healthy, youthful glow to the skin.

Facial stone therapy

The use of hot and cool stones in facial treatments has developed due to the rise in popularity of hot stone therapy. It is a specialised treatment involving basalt (hot

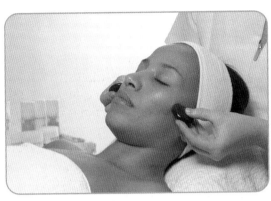
Stone therapy

stones) and marble (cool stones) in place of manual massage in a facial. A stone facial is a unique experience and helps massage the lymphatic system and create a gentle and efficient drainage.

Benefits

- Provides a deeper elimination of toxins and blockages with a lymphatic drainage massage.
- Improves skin firmness and vibrancy, while reducing redness with the hot and cold.
- Provides deeper relaxation of the muscles with the heat of the stones.
- Balances and grounds energy.
- Provides specialised techniques that can only be done by the facial therapist and not duplicated at home.
- All skin types and ages can experience it (although care needs to be taken to work with cooler stones on sensitive, inflamed skins and those clients with heart and circulatory problems).

FAQs: Facial treatments

What additional beauty therapy services could be offered at the same time as a facial?
Offer to shape or tidy the eyebrows, give an eyelash tint or incorporate a hand, foot or head massage. Remember treatments are only limited by your imagination. The main consideration is to avoid offering any service which may cause adverse effects (i.e. waxing, applying a full make-up).

I learnt a classical deep cleansing facial massage when I was training, but would like to learn additional techniques. Does this mean I need to attend another training course?
You will find once you are experienced at giving facial massage you will inevitably develop your own style of movements to suit your client's needs, and will add little touches based on your own flair and experience. However, it is always advisable to attend further training courses to extend your continuing professional development, to give you fresh ideas and inspiration, and above all to keep you up to date.

Why is it that the eye area needs careful treatment during a facial?
The skin around the eyes is extremely thin, and is therefore more sensitive to irritation and allergy.

Do I need additional training and insurance if I want to offer my clients facial electrical treatments?
Yes, you will need additional training and insurance. Training is needed on the different machines, their benefits, contraindications, treatment planning and applications. Additional insurance is required as electrical machines present a higher risk than manual facial applications.

casestudy: male skin

Ben was 29 when he first sought professional advice about his skin. He seemed very self-conscious during our first consultation, and was using his hand to cover the lower part of his face. Upon examination, Ben's skin appeared very red and inflamed from having shaved earlier that day, and was also very dehydrated with fine lines.

Ben was not only concerned about how sore his skin appeared and felt, but he also felt his skin was ageing prematurely. When questioned, Ben said his use of products at home was limited to shaving gel and an aftershave lotion which made his skin sting!

Following the consultation, we booked the first treatment for the following week and I asked Ben to make his appointment later in the day so his skin was less sensitive from his morning shave. The initial treatment objective was to gently cleanse, soothe and hydrate the skin, without overstimulation.

The first treatment involved gently cleansing the skin with soft facial cloths, followed by a creamy non-abrasive exfoliator which was left on whilst warm towels were placed over the skin. The skin was then massaged with a light oil and a soothing, hydrating mask was applied to shaving zones of face to help suppress irritation and to soften and condition the skin. The mask was rinsed off with soft facial sponges and the treatment concluded with the application of a light moisturising lotion and a tab of eye gel.

This treatment plan was repeated on a monthly basis with Ben using the creamy exfoliator before shaving and the light moisturiser as an aftershave lotion for protection. I also encouraged Ben to use a gel around the eye area to help hydrate the skin and lessen the appearance of fine lines.

After about six weeks there was a considerable improvement to Ben's skin, which no longer appeared sore and inflamed, and was looking rejuvenated. Ben continues to visit the salon on a monthly basis for facials, which he maintains are now more for relaxation than for his skin condition!

The field of medical aesthetics is becoming one of the most exciting developments in the skincare industry. It is therefore vital for skincare therapists to keep abreast of the latest developments in advanced skincare and facial rejuvenation methods.

Whilst beauty or facial therapists are not trained to undertake medical aesthetic procedures, they can fulfil a vital role in raising awareness of the various procedures available.

Bio Skin Jetting

Bio Skin Jetting is a relatively new procedure designed to reduce the appearance of facial wrinkles, currently practised by beauty therapists. Bio Skin Jetting is a non-surgical procedure that is carried out without an anaesthetic. Treatments should last less than an hour, but clients may need up to five sessions at intervals of two weeks.

The practitioner inserts a thin probe into the wrinkle. This probe is agitated and is said to cause the top layer of skin to detach from the skin beneath and encourage the production of natural collagen fibres. As these fibres develop, they push the top layer of skin out, thereby reducing the appearance of the wrinkle. Skin should appear smoother and tighter, and wrinkles should fade. Bio Skin Jetting is not permanent and the effect may be reversed over time

The effects of Bio Skin Jetting aren't immediate – the wrinkle will appear as a thin red line after treatment and this may last for several days.

Botox®

Botox is a cosmetic enhancement treatment now commonly used to smooth away frown lines and wrinkles with amazing results. It was originally developed by an eye surgeon in the 1970s as a non-surgical way of treating many eye and neurological disorders.

Botox is a formulation of botulinum toxin type A. It is derived from the bacterium

119

Clostridium botulinum. This bacterium produces a protein that blocks the release of acetylcholine and relaxes muscles. Type A is just one of seven different types of botulinum toxin (A, B, C1, D, E, F, and G), and each has different properties and actions. No two of these botulinum toxins are alike.

By employing its ability to temporarily interrupt the flow of nerve messages to the muscles, Botox is now used to treat facial lines and wrinkles. It works by relaxing/paralysing specific muscles into which Botox has been injected. The muscles are prevented from contracting and this smooths out wrinkles in the overlying skin.

Pain is minimal: all that is normally felt is a tiny pinprick. Side effects are temporary and can occasionally include localised bruising, slight redness and itching of the skin and slight swelling. After treatment, the overlying skin remains smooth and unwrinkled, while the untreated facial muscles contract in a normal fashion, so facial expressions are minimally affected.

The effects of Botox are temporary and fairly short-lived. If clients want to remain wrinkle-free then new Botox injections should be scheduled every three to four months as the effects from the previous injections begin to wear off.

Botox

can help with	cannot help with
Horizontal forehead lines.	Surface skin blemishes.
'Crow's feet' around the eyes.	Sagging skin.
Lines between the eyes.	Thread veins.
Vertical 'necklace' lines on the neck.	Thin lips.
Downturned lips.	
Mild drooping of the eyebrows.	

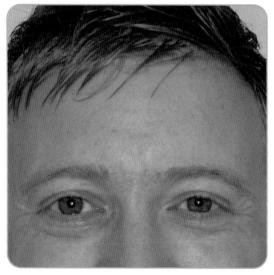

Face before Botox treatment

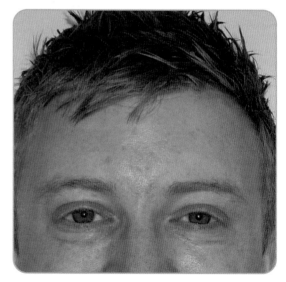

Face after Botox treatment

Chemical peels

Chemical peeling is one of the oldest cosmetic procedures in the world and was performed by ancient Egyptians, Greeks and Romans.

Today three different strengths of chemical peels are used:

- Superficial peels.
- Medium-depth peels.
- Deep peels.

> Note Beauty or facial/skincare therapists should only carry out chemical peeling treatments that involve dead and not live layers of the skin. Peeling of the *live* layers lies within the remit of a dermatologist or plastic surgeon. Advanced training and certification is required in order to carry out chemical peels safely and effectively.

Superficial peels

Superficial peeling removes only the dead cells of the epidermis and could be more properly referred to as exfoliation. Chemicals commonly used for this type of peel are alpha hydroxy acids.

Alpha hydroxy acid peels

The use of higher concentrations of alpha hydroxy acids (AHAs) in salon treatments is becoming more popular. AHA peels may be performed in conjunction with homecare programmes to treat many skin conditions such as acne-prone skin, ageing skins, sun damage, dehydration, hyperpigmentation and clogged pores.

Most salon AHA exfoliation treatments are a 15 to 30 per cent solution of alpha hydroxy acid in a gel formulation (glycolic acid being the most commonly used AHA).

Beta hydroxy peels

Salicylic acid belongs to the new generation of products for improving the appearance of ageing skin. A superior exfoliant for ageing, sun-damaged skin, salicylic acid reduces the appearance of fine lines and wrinkles and improves overall facial texture without the irritations associated with the alpha hydroxy, glycolic acid.

Medium-depth peels

These are carried out by dermatologists or cosmetic surgeons. They essentially remove the entire epidermis and can vary in the depth of dermal tissue removed.

Trichloracetic acid (TCA) is the chemical commonly used for this type of peel. TCA peels are uncomfortable during the process, but afterwards there is no discomfort and it takes about 10–12 days to heal from a good TCA peel. A TCA peel usually results in a smooth, even skin.

Deep peels

These are medical surgical peels which use a highly acidic chemical called phenol to remove tissue well into the papillary dermis. This type of peel is usually reserved for deeply wrinkled skin and skin that has been severely photo-damaged.

Dermal fillers

A dermal filler is a substance that is injected beneath lines in the skin, in order to fill the space that is causing a hollow or line to be noticeable, and can help to restore the skin to its former youthful, fuller appearance.

As the skin ages it loses some of its collagen and fat which are the materials that prevent the skin from sagging. This means that the skin becomes wrinkled. Fillers are injected into the deeper layers of the skin to plump out lines and wrinkles.

Not all lines and wrinkles are caused in the same way and therefore not all are suitable for this form of treatment. The areas which are most suitable for treatment with fillers are those around the mouth (lipstick or smoker's lines) and the nasolabial lines (those which run from the base of the nose to the corners of the mouth). Occasionally lines around the eyes may be suitable for treatment, often in combination with Botox (frown lines and 'crow's feet').

Dermal fillers

can help with	cannot help with
Lines in the forehead and eye area.	Neck lines.
Definition of the lips.	Lines from eye bags.
Sunken scars.	Lines caused by repetitive muscle action ('crow's feet').
Nasolabial folds.	

Fillers come in different thicknesses. In general, the thicker the filler product, the deeper it will be injected into the dermal layer of the skin. This helps to plump out fine to deep lines and wrinkles.

There are many different brand names of dermal fillers. However, in the UK the two most widely used products that these brands are based on are collagen and hyaluronic acid. In the UK, hyaluronic acid based products are more common. Leading brands include Restylane®, Perlane®. Matridex®, Matridur® and Hydrafill®.

Results from the treatment can been seen immediately. The gels used in facial smoothing gradually break down after nine to twelve months. Lip enhancements last for six to twelve months. Most patients who choose to have top-ups do so at the time when they feel the effect starting to wear off, that is any time between six and twelve months. Without a top-up the skin will gradually return to what it looked like before the treatment.

Collagen

Collagen is a naturally occurring protein found within the skin structure, that provides support, texture and suppleness. This treatment replaces the skin's natural collagen with a form of injectable collagen, which is patented under the trade names Zyderm® and Zyplast®, and is derived from purified bovine collagen.

Collagen injections may be used to treat many facial areas including frown lines, 'crow's feet' and lipstick lines. It is very good for improving the lips' natural shape and outline.

The primary risks of collagen injection include an allergic reaction to the collagen, infection, abscess formation and lumpiness in the treated area. While most patients do not experience these complications, it is important to understand them prior to undergoing collagen injections. Suitability for the treatment is assessed by full consultation and medical history. To avoid an allergic reaction a skin test using a tiny quantity of collagen is performed prior to treatment.

A collagen replacement therapy treatment takes approximately 30-40 minutes and lasts for four to six months depending on the individual's reabsorption rate.

Hyaluronic acid gel fillers

Restylane® is made from hyaluronic acid, a naturally occurring substance in the body that depletes as we age. Hyaluronic acid is one of the very few substances that is identical in all species and tissue types, thus it can be used in many medical applications. As it contains no animal-derived ingredients, no skin test is needed.

Treatments rarely take longer than 30 minutes and results are instantaneous. Once injected, Restylane products naturally integrate into the surrounding tissue allowing the free passage of cells and vital nutrients.

The amount of time the effects last can vary. It very much depends on factors such as age, lifestyle, structure and condition of the skin, degree of correction required and area treated. Most patients choose to have a further treatment within a year, however with lip treatments follow-up may be required within six months.

The safety of Restylane is clinically proven and documented.

Poly-L-lactic acid

Sculptra® is a truly unique facial enhancement that can help a person look years younger. It is a synthetic injectable material known as 'poly-L-lactic acid'. Poly-L-lactic acid is biocompatible (a material that does not harm

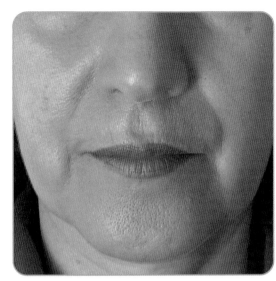
Face before dermal filler

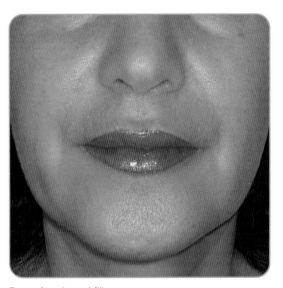
Face after dermal filler

the body) and biodegradable (able to be broken down by the body). Poly-L-lactic acid has been widely used for many years in dissolvable stitches, soft tissue implants, and other types of implants.

Sculptra is injected below the surface of the skin in the area of fat loss, and provides a gradual increase in skin thickness. Visible

123

results appear within the first few treatment sessions. Sculptra contains skin-smoothing microparticles to help lift and smooth sagging skin, severe wrinkles, creases, dark circles and scars. Although it will not correct the underlying cause of the facial fat loss, it will improve the appearance of the skin. No skin testing is required prior to use.

The results from the treatment are not immediate. After the first treatment, it may appear that Sculptra has worked immediately because of swelling from the injections and the water used to dilute Sculptra. In a few days, when the swelling goes down and the water is absorbed by the body, you may look as you did before your treatment. Several treatment sessions are needed to allow Sculptra to gradually correct the depression in the skin. The number of treatment sessions will vary from client to client; those with severe facial fat loss may require three to six treatments.

Treatment results will differ for each person. In a clinical study, the results in many patients lasted for up to two years after the first treatment session. Touch-up treatments may be needed to maintain the desired effect.

Isolagen®

Isolagen is a revolutionary process which uses a sample of your skin to replicate your own collagen producing cells (fibroblasts). Isolagen is also known as 'autologous collagen' or 'autologous cell therapy', meaning that it uses your own cells to reduce wrinkles and can result in smoother looking skin, improved texture, tone and resiliency. The Isolagen laboratory will grow millions of your cells which will be placed back into your skin where they will work to improve the skin's appearance.

Step 1

An Isolagen physician takes tiny skin samples from behind your ear under local anaesthetic. Your samples are specially packaged and sent immediately to the Isolagen laboratory where they are given a unique barcode, ensuring and protecting your identity throughout the entire process. From these samples the cells develop exponentially: their number doubles every time the cells divide. It takes time and expense to grow millions of your own fibroblast cells.

After up to twelve weeks, the fibroblasts number tens of millions and are ready to be injected into your skin. This timing will depend upon how fast your own cells grow: everyone is unique in this respect.

Steps 2 and 3

Your first treatment can be scheduled twelve weeks after your skin samples have been sent to the laboratory. The treatment recommended by physicians involves two initial sessions of injections spaced 30 to 45 days apart.

Results

Patients and physicians have reported a gradual improvement in skin texture, tone and elasticity. Typically, you may start to see results two months after your treatment in the form of better, more unified skin, a softening of fine lines and wrinkles, and scars could become smoother.

Light rejuvenation therapy

Light rejuvenation therapy is designed to reduce wrinkles and fine lines, and areas of uneven pigmentation.

> Note This treatment should only be carried out by a trained operator in an establishment registered by the Healthcare Commission.

Light rejuvenation treatments use lasers, intense pulsed light or light heat energy systems. These treatments are 'non-ablative'. This means that they affect the middle or dermal layer of the skin without causing too much damage to the top layer of the skin. The treatment works by stimulating the dermal layer of the skin to produce more collagen, which 'plumps out' fine lines or wrinkles.

The eyes must be protected with specially designed goggles during the treatment. Different light-based systems will work differently on different skin types. An initial course of treatments may be needed to achieve the desired effect, and a further treatment every six months may be necessary to maintain this effect. Clients should make sure that their chosen clinic has a light-based system which can achieve the result they want for their skin and pigmentation type.

Laser skin resurfacing

The objective of laser resurfacing treatments is to reduce blemishes, fine lines, uneven pigmentation and scars.

> Note This treatment should only be carried out by a trained operator in an establishment registered by the Healthcare Commission.

These treatments are 'ablative'. This means that the laser beam will remove the top layer of the skin. When the skin heals and grows back it should do so without the blemishes, wrinkles and scars which were previously there. A local anaesthetic may be used for the treatment and the eyes must be protected with specially designed goggles. The treatment may take up to 30 minutes, and there may be some pain.

The skincare regime in the week following the procedure is demanding and it is extremely important that it is adhered to rigidly. The regime will consist of rigorous cleansing of the skin every two to three hours initially and thorough moisturising using prescribed products. The skin will remain red for approximately six months after treatment and must be protected from the sun for a year.

Laser skin resurfacing can remove acne scars, birthmarks, sun damage and other skin blemishes. Clients should make sure that their chosen clinic has a light-based system which can achieve the result they want for their skin and pigmentation type.

Microdermabrasion

Microdermabrasion is a mechanical exfoliation of the top layer of the skin (stratum corneum) through the use of a machine that fires crystals (aluminium salts, sodium chloride or sodium bicarbonate) over the skin whilst the dead skin cells are removed using suction. It is basically like an ultra-advanced facial scrub.

Generally the more powerful machines are made available to dermatologists and other medical practitioners, while the less powerful machines are used by beauty therapists and aestheticians.

Microdermabrasion requires no special skin preparation, other than cleansing with a gentle soap-free cleanser. During treatment, there is a sensation of very superficial scraping, similar to when using a loofah or when carrying out mild skin exfoliation. The treatment usually takes approximately 30 minutes and is usually given at least once or twice a month. Results should be evident straight away and the skin should look brighter and pinker. Clients may apply make-up and go out and about immediately after treatment, if required.

Microdermabrasion

can help with	cannot help with
Brightening dull skin.	Deeper scarring.
Areas of irregular pigmentation.	Spider or thread veins.
Dark, superficial scarring.	Lumps on the skin.
Small shallow scars.	Deeper pigmentation/dark patches.
Areas of comedones, milia, and small acne lesions.	

FAQs: Non-surgical methods

I have heard you can buy Botox creams. Are these effective?

In a word, 'No'! The molecules are too large to be able to penetrate the skin and therefore cannot work effectively in a cream form.

Lots of my clients are interested in having Botox. How can you tell if a client is a suitable candidate?

The best thing to do is to observe the client's muscles at rest. If the lines are visible at rest and increase the appearance of ageing then Botox is recommended. However, if the client has slight lines when they smile and frown and none at rest then it is best for them to wait until a later time.

I have a client who has recently had Botox injections in her forehead. Is it safe for her to continue having facial treatments?

Botox starts to work between four and seven days following treatment. It is therefore best to avoid any form of facial application until at least seven days have elapsed, and by this stage any swelling or inflammation that may have resulted from the injection will have subsided. Provided there are no complications salon treatments may be safely resumed.

I have a client who had eyelift surgery (blepharoplasty) just over a month ago. How soon after facial surgery is it possible for her to recommence her facial treatments? Are there any precautions I should take?

It is important never to commence facial treatment of a post-surgical client without the approval of the cosmetic surgeon (generally salon treatments may resume approximately three to four weeks following surgery). Facial treatment should be avoided whilst sutures are still in the skin. It is important to be extremely gentle with all facial procedures and use of products (avoiding anything harsh and abrasive) following surgery, being especially careful to support the skin fully to avoid dragging the tissue around the eyes. Mild massage may be carried out around the lids after they have healed to help dissipate the discoloration from bruising and swelling.

What advice would you offer clients who are considering having cosmetic facial surgery?

Advise them to seek out as much information as possible on the procedures available and the risks. A good source of helpful advice is on the website www.dh.gov.uk 'Considering a surgical or non-surgical procedure?' Always advise a client to seek the help of a cosmetic surgeon who has been recommended by their GP, or other practitioner, and ask to see examples of previous patients' treatments. Above all, it is important to encourage clients to be honest and realistic about their expectations and to take time to discuss the procedure fully before committing themselves.

non-surgical methods of advanced skincare

where to go from here

The official national training organisation for the hair and beauty industry

🖎 Habia
Oxford House
Sixth Avenue
Sky Business Park
Robin Hood Airport

Doncaster
DN9 3GG
Tel: 08452 306080
www.habia.org.uk

Awarding bodies of professional qualifications in facial massage and skincare/beauty therapy

🖎 VTCT
Third Floor
Eastleigh House
Upper Market Street
Eastleigh
Hampshire
SO50 9FD
www.vtct.org.uk

🖎 City & Guilds
1 Giltspur Street
London
EC1A 9DD
Tel: 020 7294 2800
Email: enquiry@cityandguilds.com

BTEC/Edexcel
Edexcel Customer Service
One90 High Holborn
London
WC1V 7BH
Tel: 0870 240 9800
www.edexcel.org.uk

Confederation of International Beauty
Therapy and Cosmetology
CIBTAC Administration Office
Meteor Court
Barnett Way
Gloucester
GL4 3GG
Tel: +44 (0) 1452 623114
Fax: +44 (0) 1452 611724
Email: jane@babtac.com

ITEC
2nd floor, Chiswick Gate
598–608 Chiswick High Road
London
W4 5RT
Tel: +44 (0)20 8994 4141
Fax: +44 (0)20 8994 7880
Email: info@itecworld.co.uk
www.itecworld.co.uk

The Guild of Professional Beauty
Therapists
Guild House
320 Burton Road
Derby
DE23 6AF
Tel: 0870 000 4242
Fax: 0870 000 4247
www.beautyguild.com

Professional associations

The Federation of Holistic Therapists
(FHT)
18 Shakespeare Business Centre
Hathaway Close
Eastleigh
Hampshire
SO50 4SR
Membership Office:
Tel: 0870 420 2022
Fax: 023 8062 4399
Email: info@fht.org.uk
www.fht.org.uk

British Association of Beauty Therapy and
Cosmetology (BABTAC)
Meteor Court
Barnett Way
Gloucester
GL4 3GG
www.babtac.com

Embody
P O Box 6955
Towcester
NN12 6WZ
Tel: 0870 201 1912
www.EmbodyProfessional.com

Professional publications

❧ Professional Beauty
3rd Floor
Broadway House
2–6 Fulham Broadway
London
SW6 1AA
Tel: 020 7610 3001
info@professionalbeauty.co.uk

❧ Health and Beauty Salon Magazine
Reed Business Information
Quadrant House
The Quadrant
Sutton
Surrey SM2 5AS
Tel: 020 8652 3500
www.reedbusiness.co.uk

Product and equipment manufacturers

For a comprehensive list of suppliers (skincare, equipment, etc.) visit:

1 ww.beautybuyer.co.uk
2 Beautyguild Suppliers Guide:
www.beautyguild.com

3 Training DVDs by Helen McGuinness:
www.amazon.co.uk

Association contacts for information about cosmetic procedures

❧ British Association of Dermatologists
19 Fitzroy Square
London
WIT 6EH
www.bad.org.uk

❧ British Association of Aesthetic Plastic Surgeons
The Royal College of Surgeons
35–43 Lincoln's Inn Fields
London
WC2A 3PN
www.baaps.co.uk

For an A–Z of cosmetic surgery and non-surgical cosmetic procedures visit the Department of Health's website: www.dh.gov.uk

The Healthcare Commission

In April 2004, the Healthcare Commission took over responsibility for regulating and inspecting the independent (private and voluntary) healthcare sector, which was previously the responsibility of the National Care Standards Commission (NCSC). This includes establishments using laser and intense pulse light systems for non-invasive cosmetic procedures.

There are offices in London, Bristol, Leeds, Manchester, Nottingham and Solihull.

London (Head Office)
Finsbury Tower
103–105 Bunhill Row
London
EC1Y 8TG
Tel: 020 7448 9200
www.healthcarecommission.org.uk

glossary

Ablative: a term used to describe a procedure that removes the top layer of the skin

Adipose tissue: type of tissue containing fat cells, found in the subcutaneous layer of skin

Aesthetics: branch of anatomical science that deals with the overall health and well-being of the skin

Alpahydroxy acids (AHAs): a group of naturally occurring fruit acids. Used in cosmetic products as exfoliants, moisturisers and emollients

Alcohol: antiseptic and solvent used in perfumes, lotions and astringents

Allergic reaction: a disorder in which the body becomes hypersensitive to a particular allergen

Ampoule: a specialised product of highly concentrated active ingredients in a sealed vial

Antioxidants: substances (such as vitamin E) that protect the body through counteracting the damaging effects of free radical activity

Asthma: a condition producing attacks of shortness of breath and difficulty in breathing due to spasm or swelling of the bronchial tubes

Astringent: a liquid that helps remove excess oil from the skin

Ayurvedic facial massage: a form of massage using ancient Ayurvedic principles and marma point massage to help balance the client's subtle energies or dosha

Basal cell layer (stratum germinativum): deepest and innermost of the five layers of the epidermis

Bell's palsy: a disorder of the seventh cranial nerve (facial nerve) that results in paralysis on one side of the face

BioSkinJetting: a relatively new non-surgical procedure to reduce the appearance of facial wrinkles

Botox: a cosmetic treatment commonly used to smooth away frown lines and wrinkles

Cabi (hot): machine for heating towels used in steam treatments

Ceramides: naturally occurring lipids contributing to the moisturisation of the skin

Chemical peel: a cosmetic procedure which helps improve the skin's appearance when wrinkles or scarring are present

Clear layer: (stratum lucidum) epidermal layer below the most superficial layer

Coenzyme Q-10: thought to be an effective antioxidant; tends to be added to skin treatment creams

Collagen: a naturally occurring protein found within the skin structure providing support, texture and suppleness

Comedogenic: term used to describe an ingredient which may increase follicular blockages and hence the formation of comedones

Comedone: a collection of sebum, keratinised cells and wastes accumulating in the entrance of a hair follicle

Crow's feet: wrinkles at the outer corner of the eye

Cyst: an abnormal sac containing liquid or a semi-solid substance

Dehydration: a lack of moisture in the intercellular system of the skin

Dermal filler: a substance that is injected into the skin, in order to fill the space that is causing a hollow or line to be noticeable

Dermis: deeper layer of the skin found below the epidermis

Desincrustation: a deep cleansing treatment (chemical cleanse) to soften skin and remove hardened sebum and cell debris

Desquamation: the shedding of dead skin cells from the horny layer

Detergent: main type of surfactant used in skincare products

Eczema: mild to chronic inflammatory skin condition characterised by itchiness, redness and the presence of small blisters

Effleurage: light, even, stroking movements, which prepare the tissues for deeper massage and link up other movements in the facial sequence

Elastin: protein in the dermis, which helps contribute to the skin's elasticity

Emollients: fatty substances with a lubricating action which lie on the skin's surface, helping to prevent dehydration and increase water retention in the epidermis

Emulsifier: a compound added to an emulsion to help the drops to disperse, thereby allowing the separate ingredients to mix together and stabilise the mixture

Emulsion: oil and water blended together as one substance by the use of an emulsifier

Epidermis: outermost, superficial layer of the skin

Epilepsy: neurological disorder, which makes the individual susceptible to recurrent and temporary seizures

Erythema: reddening of the skin due to the dilation of blood capillaries just below the epidermis

Exfoliation: removal of dead skin cells from the outermost layer of the epidermis

Facial stone therapy: a specialised treatment using basalt (hot stones) and marble (cool stones) in place of manual massage in a facial

Fatty acids: lubricant ingredients derived from plant oils or animal fats

Fatty esters: emollients produced from fatty acids and alcohols

Fitzpatrick Scale: a scale used to measure the skin type's ability to tolerate sun exposure

Folliculitis: a bacterial infection of the hair follicles of the skin

Galvanic: a constant direct current used in facial electrical treatments

Glycolic acid: an alpha hydroxy acid derived from sugar cane

Granular layer (stratum granulosum): layer of epidermis linking the living cells of the epidermis (basal and prickle cell layers) to the dead cells above

High frequency: an alternating current which passes through the skin to produce a heating and stimulating effect

Horny layer (stratum corneum): most superficial, outer layer of the skin consisting of dead, flattened, keratinised cells

Humectants: ingredients that are used to attract water to the skin's surface

Hyaluronic acid: a moisturiser that occurs naturally in the dermis

Hyperkeratosis: a horny overgrowth of skin cells

Hyperpigmentation: an excess of pigment resulting in brown discolouration/darkening of the skin from the overproduction of melanin

Hypopigmentation: less than the normal melanin production, or the absence of pigmentation, resulting in white, colourless areas of skin

Iontophoresis: the introduction of water soluble substances deep into the skin for maximum benefit

Isolagen: a rejuvenation treatment for the skin using a small sample of your own skin to reproduce collagen producing cells

Laser skin resurfacing: a procedure used to reduce blemishes, fine lines, uneven pigmentation and scars

Light rejuvenation treatments: lasers, intense pulsed light or light heat energy systems to help to reduce wrinkles, fine lines and uneven pigmentation

Lipids: fats

Liposomes: tiny hollow spheres of lipids (fats), which are filled with active ingredients

Medical aesthetics: the integration of surgical cosmetic procedures with aesthetics

Microcurrent: an electrical facial contour lifting treatment which works by re-programming the muscle fibres

Microdermabrasion: exfoliation of the top layer of the skin using a machine that fires crystals over the skin whilst the dead skin cells are removed by suction

Migraine: specific form of headache, usually unilateral (one side of the head), associated with nausea or vomiting and visual disturbances

Oedema: an abnormal swelling of body tissues due to an accumulation of tissue fluid. May be local (as with an injury or inflammation), or pre-menstrual (subcutaneous oedema), or may be more general as in heart or kidney disease (medical oedema)

Panthenol: a substance that is readily converted into vitamin B5 when applied topically to the skin; aids tissue repair

Papillary layer: most superficial layer of dermis, situated above reticular layer

Papule: a small raised elevation on the skin, less than 1 cm in diameter, which may be red in colour

Peptides: these are chemically derived from amino acids and are used in advanced skincare formulas

Petrissage: a term used in massage to describe a range of kneading movements that stimulate the underlying tissues

Photoageing: the process by which the skin undergoes accelerated ageing after ultraviolet exposure

Preservatives: chemical agents that inhibit the growth of micro-organisms in product formulations

Prickle cell layer (stratum spinosum): binding and transitional layer between the stratum granulosum and the stratum germinativum

Pustule: an infected papule, which has a head with a white or yellow centre which contains pus

Reticular fibres: fibres found in the reticular layer of dermis which help to maintain the skin's tone, strength and elasticity

Reticular layer: deepest layer of the dermis, situated below the papillary layer

Retinoic acid (tretinoin): derivative of vitamin A, used to refine the skin, alter collagen production and reduce the appearance of wrinkles

Rosacea: a chronic inflammatory disease of the face in which the skin appears abnormally red

Sebaceous gland: oil-producing glands that are attached to hair follicles, most common on the face and upper body

Seborrhoea: an excessive secretion of sebum by the sebaceous glands

Sebum: the skin's natural moisturising factor (oil)

Serum: concentrates of active ingredients, designed to act as 'intensive correctors' for a range of skin types and conditions

Solvents: substances such as water or alcohol that dissolve other ingredients

Subcutaneous layer: a thick layer of connective tissue found below the dermis

Surfactants: chemicals that reduce the surface tension between the skin's surface and the product to aid the distribution of the product across the skin's surface

Tapotement: a term used to describe percussion movements in massage, for example tapping and/or slapping the tissues

Vibrations: rapid shaking movements produced by the fingers or thumbs in massage

Wood's Lamp: type of magnifying lamp used to carry out a more in-depth skin analysis

135

index